Ethics and Animals

In this fresh and comprehensive introduction to animal ethics, Lori Gruen weaves together poignant and provocative case studies with discussions of ethical theory, urging readers to engage critically and to reflect empathetically on our treatment of other animals. In clear and accessible language, Gruen provides a survey of the issues central to human–animal relations and a reasoned new perspective on current key debates in the field. She analyzes and explains a range of theoretical positions and poses challenging questions that directly encourage readers to hone their ethical-reasoning skills and to develop a defensible position about their own practices. Her book will be an invaluable resource for students in a wide range of disciplines, including ethics, environmental studies, veterinary science, women's studies, and the emerging field of animal studies, and is an engaging account of the subject for general readers with no prior background in philosophy.

LORI GRUEN teaches Philosophy and Feminist, Gender, and Sexuality Studies at Wesleyan University in Connecticut, where she also directs the Ethics in Society Project. She has published widely on topics in practical ethics and animal ethics.

Ethics and Animals

An Introduction

LORI GRUEN

Wesleyan University

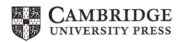

CAMBRIDGE
UNIVERSITY PRESS

CAMBRIDGE
UNIVERSITY PRESS

University Printing House, Cambridge CB2 8BS, United Kingdom

Cambridge University Press is part of the University of Cambridge.

It furthers the University's mission by disseminating knowledge in the pursuit of education, learning and research at the highest international levels of excellence.

www.cambridge.org
Information on this title: www.cambridge.org/9780521888998

First published 2011
6th printing 2014

Printed in the United States of America by Sheridan Books, Inc.

A catalog record for this publication is available from the British Library

Library of Congress Cataloging in Publication data
Gruen, Lori.
Ethics and animals : an introduction / Lori Gruen.
    p.   cm. – (Cambridge applied ethics)
Includes bibliographical references and index.
ISBN 978-0-521-88899-8
1. Animal welfare – Moral and ethical aspects.   2. Animal rights.   I. Title.
HV4708.G78   2011
179'.3 – dc22   2010041515

ISBN 978-0-521-88899-8 Hardback
ISBN 978-0-521-71773-1 Paperback

For Maggie

Contents

viii   Contents

Acknowledgments

It is through my own early exposure to animal ethics that I started to think seriously about pursuing philosophy professionally. I owe a great deal of thanks to my original teachers, who are now dear friends – Dale Jamieson and Peter Singer. My path to becoming a philosopher was punctuated by a decision to try to change attitudes about animals directly. I left graduate school during the early days of the animal rights movement and spent a number of years organizing against various forms of animal exploitation, becoming involved in exciting activist campaigns. I worked shoulder to shoulder with some incredible, inspiring people, too many to list here, but I particularly want to thank Chas Chiodo, Ken Knowles, and Vicki Miller. Over the years I have had the great pleasure to work with people who have devoted themselves to caring for animals, and in addition to allowing me to get my hands dirty they have also helped me to understand animals' interests better. I am particularly indebted to Linda Brent and Amy Fultz at Chimp Haven in Keithville, Louisiana and Patti Ragan at the Center for Great Apes in Wachula, Florida.

I have presented some of the ideas that are discussed in this book in many different places over the years. I thank audiences at Princeton University, Yale Law School, and Wellesley College for talking through some of the ideas in Chapters 1, 2, and 5 with me. I have taught animal ethics in my classes at five different universities and colleges and I am grateful to all of the students on those courses. Special thanks are owed to the students in my Humans–Animals–Nature classes at Wesleyan University in the spring 2008 and the fall 2009 with whom I worked through the material that became this book. They will undoubtedly see their objections and concerns in these pages. Special thanks to Micah Fearing, Dan Fischer, Megan Hughes, Mark Lee, and Dan Schniedewind for specific comments on some of the chapters. Thanks to Mollie Laffin-Rose for research assistance and Tyler Wuthmann for help with references. My friends at Wesleyan University in Middletown and Fresh Yoga in New Haven have provided very different, but much appreciated, support. I am so thankful to Hilary Gaskin of Cambridge University Press for seeing the need for this book and keeping me on track. I am particularly indebted to Valerie Tiberius, J. D. Walker, Kristen Olsen, and especially Robert C. Jones for providing me with detailed feedback on earlier drafts of the chapters that follow.

My deepest gratitude goes to the individual animals who have inspired, amused, and comforted me and with whom I have had rich and life-altering relationships – my late feline companions Tootie, Jason, Jeremy, Camus, and the inimical Eldridge Recatsner; my late canine companions Dooley and Buddy; and my special chimpanzee friends living in sanctuary at Chimp Haven: Sarah, Sheba, Emma, Harper, Ivy, Keeli, and Darrell. Darrell and Buddy passed away while I was writing this book, but remembering their strong personalities and courage kept me going. My beloved canine companion Maggie and her dog Fuzzy have been by my side (more accurately, at my feet) as I have been working away at the computer. Maggie was particularly tolerant of my stress as the deadline for submitting the book approached. She has helped me through many losses and challenges; her loyalty and care for me is a model of virtuous ethical attention. I dedicate this book to her.

Abbreviations

AETA	Animal Enterprise Terrorism Act
ALF	Animal Liberation Front
AMC	Argument from Marginal Cases
ASL	American Sign Language
AWA	Animal Welfare Act
AZA	Association of Zoos and Aquariums
CAFO	concentrated animal feeding operation
EPA	Environmental Protection Agency
FBI	Federal Bureau of Investigation
HSUS	Humane Society of the United States
IACUC	Institutional Animal Care and Use Committee
IPCC	Intergovernmental Panel on Climate Change
IUCN	International Union for Conservation of Nature
MRSA	methicillin-resistant *Staphylococcus aureus*
NSUT	non-speciesist utilitarian test
PETA	People for the Ethical Treatment of Animals
PTSD	post-traumatic stress disorder
SCIs	spinal cord injuries
SHAC	Stop Huntingdon Animal Cruelty
ToM	theory of mind
UNEP	United Nations Environment Program
USDA	United States Department of Agriculture
USGS	United States Geological Survey
WWF	World Wildlife Fund

Preface

Explorations of our ethical relations to other animals go back to antiquity, but it wasn't until the 1970s, in the wake of social justice struggles for racial and gender equality, that animal ethics was taken up seriously by philosophers and other theorists and the modern animal rights movement was born. When I first started working on animal ethics it was still somewhat on the fringe of both the academy and society more generally, so it is really exciting for me to see a whole academic field emerge, called "animal studies," and to watch animal ethics become more mainstream. So much theoretical work has been done in the last ten or so years, that I think it is safe to say we are now in the "second wave" of animal ethics.

Introductory texts should try to present all reasonable sides of an issue and I believe I have done that in the pages that follow. However, because I have been thinking, writing, and teaching about animal ethics for over two decades I have well-worked-out views on the issues I present in this book and, as I tell my students, it would be disingenuous to pretend otherwise, so I do not try to hide my considered judgments. My commitment is obvious – other animals deserve our moral attention and their lives matter – and this is the perspective that shapes this book. I do not take one particular philosophical position and explore it in depth in this volume, however. Rather, given that there are competing ethical issues in play and many conflicts of values that are not obviously or readily resolvable, I try to highlight the ethical complexity of our interactions with and obligations to other animals as well as to point to some of the limitations of popular ethical approaches. Even among those who believe that animals matter, there is disagreement. I have explored some of the disagreement within animal ethics here, but of course I couldn't cover everything. Many will disagree with the arguments I present, but one of my goals is to provide readers with enough arguments and information to help them to develop their own views that they then feel confident defending.

There is a tendency in almost any ethical discussion to flatten out or over-simplify opposing views and to caricature opponents. This is certainly the case in discussions of animal ethics. For example, those opposed to research on animals often think that all of those who use animals for scientific purposes are insensitive to animals and to animal rights advocates. I have found this isn't true. Similarly, zoo advocates tend to lump everyone who opposes captivity together – as radicals who would rather all animals become extinct than subject them to imprisonment. I have found this isn't true either. It's a lot simpler to think of things as strictly dichotomous; it certainly is a lot simpler to write as if that is so, and I'm afraid I do sometimes oversimplify theoretical positions, particularly when I am trying to make a philosophical point as precisely as possible. But, in reality, most positions are much more nuanced and the people who hold various positions about animals fall along a spectrum. And, people's attitudes about other animals are not always consistent. I have friends who have dedicated their lives to protecting and rescuing some animals who also eat other animals. I know vegetarians who experiment on animals and vegans who support regularly killing animals in certain contexts. This variety makes teaching animal ethics particularly interesting. Unlike many philosophical topics, we are all implicated in the practices that I examine in this book.

I have organized the book in a way that I think is both accessible to the interested reader and helpful to those who would like to use this book in the classroom. Each chapter starts with a vignette that raises some of the ethical issues that will be explored in the chapter. I think it is particularly important in teaching and thinking about ethics that we don't allow theory to get too far removed from practice. Information about real-world ethical problems should shape our philosophical reflections, so I often seek out expert (non-philosophical) insights and knowledge about practices. Philosopher Henry Sidgwick said it best, I think:

> Our aim is to frame an ideal of the good life ... and to do this satisfactorily and completely we must have adequate knowledge of the conditions of this life in all the bewildering complexity and variety in which it is actually being lived ... we can only do this by a comprehensive and varied knowledge of the actual opportunities and limitations, the actual needs and temptations, the actually constraining customs and habits, desires, and fears ... and this knowledge a philosopher – whose personal experience is often very limited – cannot adequately attain unless he earnestly avails himself of

opportunities of learning from the experiences of [others] . . . the philosopher's practical judgment on particular problems is likely to be untrustworthy, unless it is aided and controlled by the practical judgment of others who are not philosophers.[1]

I have sought out information and "practical judgment" right up to the last minute, to keep the discussion as up to date as possible. I have also included my own experiences working with animals and the insights of people who are involved in many different aspects of the issues discussed here – e.g., those who work in labs, those who work at zoos, those who oppose the use of animals in labs, those who oppose zoos, those who care directly for animals in shelters and sanctuaries, those who study animals in the wild.

If this book is to be used as a textbook, the chapters lend themselves to being taught in quite different ways, depending on the nature of the course and the interests of the instructor. The first two chapters present the ethical arguments that are at the heart of discussions about the extent and nature of our obligations to other animals. Though these chapters are self-contained, teachers may wish to supplement these chapters with texts that explore the history of ethics, topics in animal cognition, comparative psychology, philosophy of biology, disability studies, or texts that directly challenge anthropocentrism. The remaining chapters allow for similar supplementation depending on the instructor's interest. Chapter 3 would lend itself to a larger discussion of the ethics of killing or the philosophy of food. In Chapter 4 I only touch briefly on the topic of pain, on which a great deal of interesting philosophical and scientific work has been done; veterinary medicine also has much to contribute here. There are also topics in the history and philosophy of science into which this chapter provides an entrée. Chapter 5 might be supplemented with more in-depth discussions of autonomy, political philosophy, or topics in the philosophy of mind. Chapter 6 could be the basis for a nice module on environmental philosophy and conservation biology. Chapter 7 deals with animal activism, and there is much more that might be said about legal protection for other animals as well as the relation of animal activism to other forms of social justice activism. Of course, these are just suggestions; I hope that the book is useful to those teaching animal studies from a variety of disciplinary and interdisciplinary perspectives.

---

[1] Sidgwick 1998: 20–1.

I need to make a few comments about terminology. The term "animal" has been contested as it is used in very different ways. Often it is meant to exclude humans, but, of course, humans are animals. The term is so vast, it contains so many different organisms, that it is sometimes too general a term to be very useful. To be more specific, sometimes writers, including myself, use "non-human animal" to refer to other animals. Some argue that this sets humans above other animals. To rectify this, sometimes people use the term "other than human animals," but this is rather bulky. I use "other animals" as often as makes sense. I also use "non-human animals" and just "animals" sometimes too.

Some philosophers separate the "ethical" from the "moral." I use these terms interchangeably here.

I also want to bring to your attention my use of pronouns. In gender studies, pronoun use is a particularly important topic, as the use of gender-neutral and gender-inclusive pronouns, or, more precisely, the lack of their use, have implications beyond grammar. In animals studies, the struggle is moving from "it," which refers to inanimate objects, to "he" or "she." It is tricky when it isn't clear what sex the particular individual to whom I am referring is, so sometimes I will refer to an animal whose sex I don't know as "he," sometimes as "she." Speaking of "whom," my spellcheck constantly reminds me of the error of my pronoun use in sentences in which I referred to animals as "who" rather than "that." I ignored the spellcheck.

Although I have been thinking and working on the topics I present here for many years, at times, working on this book made me very sad. We humans have done unnecessary and incredibly cruel things to other animals. While reviewing the history of animal experimentation and zoos, evaluating the current state of animal agriculture, reporting on the bushmeat crisis and rates of extinction, it occasionally felt that ethical discussion could barely scratch the surface of our entrenched callous practices, and the task of changing such practices often seems insurmountable. But, being in the presence of other animals, experiencing their incredible capacities for forgiveness, knowing remarkable people who spend their lives improving animal lives, and working with students who are eager to try to make a difference, gives me hope. Part of my hope is that this book will help readers to rethink their relationships with other animals and perhaps move you to do one thing, every day, to make the world better for all animals, human and non-human.

1 Why animals matter

In early summer 2004, off the northern coast of the North Island of New Zealand, four swimmers were suddenly surrounded by a pod of bottlenose dolphins herding them into a tight circle. The dolphins were agitated, flapping at the water, and they continuously circled the swimmers, keeping them close together for over half an hour. A lifeguard patrolling in a boat nearby saw the commotion and dove in with the swimmers to find out what was happening. While under water, he saw a great white shark, now swimming away, beneath the swimmers. Presumably, the arrival of his patrol boat had scared the shark off, but it was the dolphins who were protecting the swimmers from a shark attack until help arrived. Dr. Rochelle Constantine, from the Auckland University School of Biological Science, noted that this behavior was rare, but not unheard of. "From my understanding of the behaviour of these dolphins they certainly were acting in a way which indicated the shark posed a threat to something. Dolphins are known for helping helpless things. It is an altruistic response and bottlenose dolphins in particular are known for it."[1]

Are dolphins really altruistic? Do they think of humans as helpless things? Can they understand threats to individuals other than themselves? Do they care about other individuals, even members of different species? If dolphins care about us, should we care about them and other animals? The anecdote about dolphins saving humans from a potential shark attack generates curiosity and amazement and opens up a world of questions, many of which we will address throughout this book.

Humans have always lived with or in close proximity to other animals. Animals have worked beside us. They have hunted us, and we have hunted them. We have used them as human surrogates in scientific and medical

---

[1] www.nzherald.co.nz/nz/news/article.cfm?c_id=1&objectid=3613343.

experiments, and we have physically and genetically altered them to suit our tastes, our lifestyles, and our domestic needs. They have been the source of entertainment, inspiration, loyalty, and devotion. Non-human animals also serve a conceptual role in helping us define ourselves as human. We are not them. It is against the animal that we define humanity. Their differences from us highlight our similarity to other humans. Both the actual and the conceptual relationships humans have with other animals raise ethical questions, as do all relationships between feeling individuals. We coexist with other animals on a planet that does not have resources to sustain all of us endlessly. Many, if not all, of our decisions and actions affect not just fellow humans, but fellow animals as well. In this book we will explore a variety of ethical issues raised by the relationships humans have with other animals.

Not everyone agrees that there are ethical issues raised by our relations to animals, so we should start by examining the view that we do not have ethical responsibilities to other animals. This view – what I will call human exceptionalism – results, in part, from the way we psychologically and intellectually distance ourselves from our own animal natures and, by extension, from other animals. Our humanity is distinct from, and some even suggest, transcends, our animality. We see humans as world-builders and meaning-makers and think other animals are not. We engage in uniquely human activities, activities that elevate us above animals. Because humans are thought to occupy a separate and superior sphere, some people believe that only humans are the proper subjects of ethical concern.

This view has lofty historical antecedents. Aristotle was probably the most prominent early philosopher to argue that animals were lower on a natural hierarchy because they lacked reason. This natural hierarchy, he believed, gave those on higher rungs both the right and the responsibility to use those on the lower rungs. Later, the Stoics went a bit farther and denied that animals had any capacity for thought and existed solely to be used. As philosopher Richard Sorabji writes:

> The most extreme elaboration of the idea that animals are for man is found in the Stoics. According to Chrysippus, bugs are useful for waking us up and mice for making us put our things away carefully. Cocks have come into being for a useful purpose too: they wake us up, catch scorpions, and arouse us to battle, but they must be eaten, so there won't be more chicks than is useful. As for the pig, it is given a soul . . . of salt, to keep it fresh for us to eat.[2]

---

[2] Sorabji 1993: 199.

Early Christian theologians, with the noted exception of Francis of Assisi, also viewed animals as fundamentally distinct from humans in that they lacked souls and were here just to satisfy human ends.[3] And the "father of modern philosophy," René Descartes, is the most commonly cited proponent of the view that humans have minds and are thus ensouled beings who have moral standing, while other animals are merely bodily, mechanical creatures here for us to use as we want. For Descartes, not unlike his predecessors, animals were thought of simply as living machines who respond automatically to stimuli, unaware that anything is happening to them when they encounter such stimuli. Their lack of reason, thoughts, consciousness, and souls corresponds with their lack of moral standing. We don't have ethical relationships with alarm clocks, toasters, or cell phones and we don't have ethical relationships with other animals.

Despite their dismissive attitudes toward other animals, even these thinkers believed that there were some ethical issues raised by our interactions with them. No reflective person thinks that wanton cruelty to animals does not raise ethical concerns. In fact, it is quite common to find examples in the philosophical literature of actions involving such wanton cruelty that are thought to be unarguably wrong. If it makes sense to say it is wrong to torture a dog for fun or to burn a cat alive out of curiosity, then it appears that on some occasions other animals can appropriately be the subjects of ethical assessments. Some philosophers have suggested that the wrongness of acts of wanton cruelty does not arise from the *direct* harm the act has on the animal victims, but rather that such actions are thought to be wrong because they reflect the type of character that often allows a person to engage in unethical behavior toward humans. According to Immanuel Kant, for example, although "irrational animals" were mere things to which we have no direct duties and "with which one may deal and dispose at one's discretion," there are implications of actions toward animals for humanity. For Kant, "if a man has his dog shot, because it can no longer earn a living for him, he is by no

---

[3] Trying to articulate how animals made their way through the world without the ability to think often generated extreme philosophical contortions, as in this quote from Augustine: "Though in fact we observe that infants are weaker than the most vulnerable of the young of other animals in the control of their limbs, and in their instincts of appetition and defense, this seems designed to enhance man's superiority over other living things, on the analogy of an arrow whose impetus increases in proportion to the backward extension of the bow." *City of God*, Book XIII, Chapter 3. Thanks to Mary Jane Rubenstein for bringing this quote to my attention.

means in breach of any duty to the dog, since the latter is incapable of judgment, but he thereby damages the kindly and humane qualities in himself, which he ought to exercise in virtue of his duties to mankind."[4] According to thinkers who embrace some form of human exceptionalism, when a non-human animal is tortured, the harm to the animal is not what matters from an ethical point of view but rather the harm that reflects on the torturer and the society to which the torturer belongs.

Many in law enforcement believe that cruelty to animals is a precursor to violent crimes against humans, and some of the most notorious serial killers had an early history of animal abuse. Torturing and killing animals are also signs of antisocial psychological disorders. Consider a case of cruelty that occurred in New York City in the summer of 2009. Cheyenne Cherry, aged 17, after being arrested on animal cruelty and burglary charges, admitted in court that she let a kitten roast to death in an oven. According to newspaper reports, Cherry and a friend "ransacked a Bronx, NY apartment before putting the cat, Tiger Lily, in the oven, where it cried and scratched before dying." While leaving court, Cherry was confronted by animal protection activists holding signs protesting the killing. "It's dead, bitch!" snapped the unrepentant Cherry to the activists outside the court, while grinning widely and taking credit for stuffing the helpless kitten into a 500-degree oven. The kind of depravity that Cherry displayed raises concerns about her ability to make any moral judgments at all and her suitability for living freely in society.

Philosophers, generally known for their consistent reasoning, have not been completely consistent in their attitudes about ethics and animals. This is probably due, at least in part, to an untenable commitment to human exceptionalism. In the next section, we will explore this view in some depth to see just how it is problematic.

Analyzing human exceptionalism

There are two distinguishable claims implicit in human exceptionalism. The first is that humans are unique, humans are the only beings that do or have X (where X is some activity or capacity); and the second is that humans, by doing or having X, are superior to those that don't do or have X. The first claim raises largely empirical questions – what is this X that only we do or have,

---

[4] Kant 2001: 212.

and are we really the only beings that do or have it? The second claim raises an evaluative or normative question – if we do discover the capacity that all and only humans share, does that make humans better, or more deserving of care and concern, than others from an ethical point of view? Why does doing or having X entitle humans to exclusive moral attention? In order to evaluate the legitimacy of human exceptionalism, we will need to explore these two separate claims.

How are we different?

Let's start with the empirical questions. Surely, we are different from other animals, but can we establish what it is that makes us unique? What capacities do all humans have that other animals don't? What do we do that no other animal does?

Many candidate capacities have been proposed to distinguish humans from other animals. Solving social problems, expressing emotions, starting wars, developing culture, having sex for pleasure, and having a sense of humor are just some of the traits that were considered uniquely human at one point or another. As it turns out, none of these is uncontroversially unique to humans. All animals living in socially complex groups solve various problems that inevitably arise in such groups. Canids and primates are particularly adept at it, yet even chickens and horses are known to recognize large numbers of individuals in their social hierarchies and to maneuver within them. One of the ways that non-human animals negotiate their social environments is by being particularly attentive to the emotional states of those around them. When a conspecific is angry, for example, it is a good idea to get out of his way. Animals that develop lifelong bonds are known to suffer terribly from the death of their companions. Some will risk their own lives for their mates, while others are even said to die of sorrow. Coyotes, elephants, geese, primates, and killer whales are among the species for which profound effects of grief have been reported.[5] Recently observed elephant rampages have led some to posit that other animals are prone to post-traumatic stress, not unlike soldiers returning from war.[6] While the lives of many, perhaps most, animals in the wild are consumed with struggles for survival, aggression, and battle, there

---

[5] Bekoff 2002.   [6] Bradshaw 2009.

are some whose lives are characterized by expressions of joy, playfulness, and a great deal of laughter and sex.[7]

Studying animal behavior is a fascinating and informative way to identify both differences and similarities between our way of being in the world and the way that other animals make their ways. So much of what we observe them doing allows us to reflect on what we are doing, often to our surprise and delight. However, it isn't simply the differences and similarities in behaviors that are at the heart of human exceptionalism, but rather what underlies that behavior – the *cognitive* skills that we have and they lack. Our intelligence, many have argued, is what makes us unique. If claims of human uniqueness are to be more than trivially true – only humans have human intelligence, because only humans are human – there will need to be some capacity or set of capacities that track this unique intelligence. What might the capacities that are indicative of unique human intelligence be?

Tool use

For a long time, many thought that humans were the only creatures that had the ability to make and use tools, and it was this tool-using capacity that marked our unique intelligence. Early on it was even proposed that we be classified as *Homo faber*, "man the toolmaker," rather than *Homo sapiens*, "wise man," to highlight our particularly creative, intelligent nature.[8] The view that humans are the only animals that use tools was initially challenged in the mid-1960s when Jane Goodall made a startling discovery at her Gombe field station in Tanzania. Chimpanzees were removing leaves from twigs and using the twigs to fish for termites by inserting them into termite mounds. After creating the right tool and inserting it into the mound, a chimpanzee would carefully remove the twig once the termites had climbed on, and then promptly run the termite-coated twig through his teeth for a protein-rich meal.[9] Ethologists began observing other animals, even birds, using tools. New Caledonia crows, for example, have been observed using sticks as tools in the wild; and in a lab, an untrained female crow, presented with a pipe-like structure containing a food bucket with a handle, bent a piece of wire into a hook to retrieve the bucket from inside the pipe.[10] The species of dolphins

---

[7] Woods 2010.   [8] Napier 1964 and Oakley 1949.
[9] Goodall 1964. See also Goodall 1986.   [10] Hunt 1996. See also Weir, et al. 2002.

that saved the swimmers from a great white shark are also known to use tools. Bottlenose dolphins in Australia have been observed using sea sponges as tools. With sponges covering their beaks, they dive to the bottom of deep channels and poke their tools into the sandy ocean floor to flush out small fish dwelling there. They then drop their sponges, eat the fish, and retrieve their sponges for another round. According to the scientists studying the dolphins, they are able to sweep away much more sand when they use the sponges.[11]

As exciting as these observations are, they are usually dismissed as a true challenge to human uniqueness. The chimpanzees' termite fishing rods, the New Caledonia crows' food-fetching hooks, and dolphin fishing sponges are examples of non-human animals using simple tools. But humans develop *toolkits* that can serve different functions, and animals don't use toolkits.

Or do they?

Christopher Boesch and his colleagues observed chimpanzees first using a stone to crack a nut and then a stick to dig the edible nutmeat out. The chimpanzees were using different tools sequentially to achieve their goal. In other words, they had developed a toolkit.[12] Japanese primatologists observed chimpanzees making leaf sponges to soak up water; when the water was out of reach, the chimpanzees would push the leaf sponges into the hard-to-reach areas with sticks. Recently, chimpanzees in the Congo were observed using toolkits that consist of two kinds of sticks – a thick one to punch a hole in an ant nest and a thin, flexible one to fish for the ants. If the chimpanzees were simply to break open the nest, the ants would swarm, delivering painful bites, and the chimpanzees would have fewer ants to eat.[13] So chimpanzees combine different tools to achieve their ends.[14]

Combining tools has also been observed in crows. In a laboratory experiment conducted in New Zealand, New Caledonia crows were presented with a short stick (and a useless rock); a toolbox, into which the bird could place her beak but not her whole head, containing a longer stick; and a piece of food buried in a hole that could not be reached with the short stick but could be reached with the long stick. In order to get the food, the bird would have to use the short stick to retrieve the long stick from the toolbox and then carry the long stick to the buried food to extract it. Six out of the seven crows initially attempted to retrieve the long stick with the short stick, and four

---

[11] Mann, et al. 2008.   [12] Boesch & Boesch 1990.   [13] Sanz, et al. 2009.
[14] Sugiyama & Koman 1979.

obtained the food reward on their first try.[15] That apes and birds combine different tools to solve problems suggests that humans are not unique as tool-users.

Those who hold on to the notion that tool use is the trait that makes humans unique have come up with ever finer distinctions, some suggesting that what makes human tool use different is that humans follow cultural trends in tool-using. Then primatologists observing chimpanzees in Africa began to notice cultural variation in tool use in different locations and among different groups of chimpanzees.[16] When the directors of nine long-term chimpanzee field sights in Africa compared notes, thirty-nine behavioral patterns were identified as cultural variants, and these variations cannot be accounted for by ecological or environmental explanations. For example, one group of wild chimpanzees might crack nuts with stones while another geographically distant group might crack nuts with wood, when both stones and wood are available in both sites. Another group might not eat the nuts at all, even though they are available. Victoria Horner and her colleagues decided it might be useful to see whether or not captive chimpanzees demonstrate signs of cultural variation in tool use. Sure enough, they found that after teaching the dominant members of one group one technique for acquiring food and the dominant members of another group an alternative technique for acquiring food from the same device, the particular behavior introduced to the first group spread within that group, while the alternative foraging behavior introduced to the second group spread within that group. These results suggested that "a nonhuman species can sustain unique local cultures, each constituted by multiple traditions." The scientists concluded, "The convergence of these results with those from the wild implies a richness in chimpanzees' capacity for culture."[17]

Still not satisfied, those seeking to establish human exceptionalism suggested that making and gathering tools prior to encountering a problem is uniquely human. But those crafty crows have been observed creating particularly functional tools and then holding on to them for some time. Researchers from Oxford mounted miniature cameras on crows in their wild habitats and found that a favored tool was used over a prolonged period of time, sometimes carried in flight from one location to another.[18]

---

[15] Taylor, et al. 2007.   [16] Whiten, et al. 2001.

[17] Horner & de Waal 2009. See also Horner, et al. 2006 and Whiten, et al. 2007.

[18] Norris 2007.

Perhaps only humans use tools to plan and execute a hunt and that is what makes us unique. Planning ahead requires a type of intelligence that only humans have. Again, chimpanzees disproved a claim of human uniqueness when they were observed making and using tools to hunt. At the Fongoli research site in Senegal, Jill Pruetz reported twenty-two occasions on which ten different chimpanzees, including female chimpanzees and youngsters, used tools to hunt bushbabies (small primates). The Fongoli chimpanzees made twenty-six different spears, each requiring up to five steps to construct, including trimming the tool tip to a point.[19] The chimpanzees prepare the spears, take them to a particular area, and then jab them forcefully into tree hollows where bushbabies nest. Pruetz has even observed what appeared to be a mother teaching toolmaking and hunting techniques to her infant. As *National Geographic* reported, "Since the 1960s scientists have known that chimpanzees are able to make and use tools – behavior once thought to be an exclusively human trait. Now . . . researcher Jill Pruetz has observed tool making behavior that further blurs the line between the apes and humans."[20]

The debate about tool use has a certain dialectic structure: the proponent of human exceptionalism posits what is thought to be a behavior indicative of a cognitive skill or capacity that only humans have, and then is proven mistaken once that behavior is observed in other animals, and then posits a more refined description of the capacity and the behaviors that might reveal that capacity, only to have a behavior of that description also observed in other animals. Debates about other candidate capacities for uniqueness follow the same dialectic. Language use, for example, thought to be the exclusive domain of humans, has been subject to a debate quite similar to the one about tool use.

Language use

Although there are interesting fables about talking animals going back to the Bible, the systematic study of animal language use did not begin until the 1950s when Keith and Kathy Hayes took in an infant chimpanzee, Viki, and raised her in their home for a little over six years as a human child, a method of rearing that came to be known as cross-fostering.[21] One of the skills they

---

[19] Pruetz & Bertolani 2007.   [20] Pruetz 2007.

[21] In the early 1930s, the Kelloggs raised an infant chimpanzee, Gua, with their son Donald, for a nine-month period to chart comparative developmental milestones and did attempt

hoped to teach Viki was to speak. By manipulating her lips and blocking her nose, they were able to get her to say "mama," "papa," "up," and "cup," but none of these words was ever uttered very clearly. Viki came to understand many spoken words even though she herself was never able to speak any. Viki died of pneumonia when she was only six and a half years old and that particular cross-fostering study ended. Only later did it become apparent that chimpanzee vocal anatomy is quite different from that of humans, making it impossible for chimpanzees to "speak" as humans do.

While human anatomy does make us unique in our ability to speak, not all humans do speak. Those who are deaf, for example, often communicate with gestures, and their sign language allows many who do not speak to communicate in complex ways. The fact that non-verbal humans use gestural language inspired Allen and Beatrix Gardner to undertake an investigation to determine whether chimpanzees could communicate using American Sign Language (ASL). Since chimpanzees and humans have similar hand dexterity, the Gardners, in the 1960s, began a cross-fostering project to teach chimpanzees sign language. The first chimpanzee to use ASL was Washoe, who learned an estimated 200 words. This was widely recognized as a remarkable achievement. But what was even more impressive was that Washoe combined the signs she learned in novel ways to communicate new ideas. For example, Washoe referred to watermelon as "candy fruit" and when she saw a swan for the first time she signed "water bird." She also taught her adopted son Loulis to communicate using ASL. Roger Fouts, who was a graduate student of the Gardners and eventually took over the research they began, conducted a five-year study in which only chimpanzees, but no humans, could use ASL in front of the young chimpanzee Loulis. By the end of the five-year period, Loulis was using seventy signs that he had learned from Washoe and other signing chimpanzees in their group – Dar, Moja, and Tatu.[22] The chimpanzees were not only using language, but they were also communicating among themselves with it and teaching it to their own kind.

There was a great deal of enthusiasm about teaching language to apes during the 1960s and 70s. During that time, Koko the gorilla began learning sign

to observe language use. Given that Gua was aged seven and a half months when the study began, and Donald was ten months, the results in terms of language use were not particularly meaningful. What was observed was primarily babbling and other guttural vocalizations. Kellogg & Kellogg 1933.

[22] See Gardner & Gardner 1989 and Fouts 1998.

language near Stanford University in California and was also able to combine words in spontaneous ways. Chantek, an orangutan who was taught sign language at the University of Tennessee before moving to Zoo Atlanta, mastered 150 signs. And there was Nim Chimpsky, born at the Institute of Primate Studies in Norman, Oklahoma, a laboratory where dozens of chimpanzees were taught to use sign language. Nim was sent to New York City where he was initially cross-fostered in an Upper West Side brownstone and trained in ASL at Columbia University under the skeptical eye of Herbert Terrace.[23] After learning approximately 150 signs, Nim was sent back to Oklahoma while Terrace and his students studied videotapes and data collected from their work with the young chimpanzee. Terrace concluded that even though Nim was trained in ways similar to Washoe, Nim's use of signs was not the same as using sign language. It lacked grammar of the kind that humans use in communicating via language. In addition, he suggested that many of the signs that Nim used, and the ways in which he ordered signs, were mere responses to cues being given by trainers or trained responses based on past successes, but they were not sentences.[24] At his most skeptical, Terrace claimed that Nim did not actually understand the meaning of the signs he was using.

This deflationary conclusion – that the kind of communication the great apes were engaged in was not really language because it lacked grammar – provided relief to proponents of human exceptionalism. However, ape researchers and the apes themselves had more to say on the matter. Sarah, a chimpanzee whose cognitive capacities were probably the most studied of all chimpanzees, used magnetic symbols representing familiar objects to communicate with researchers. If Sarah wanted an apple (or any other item not immediately present), she would place the symbol for apple on the magnetic board in addition to symbols indicating that she wanted her interlocutor to give the apple to her. The human interlocutor could rearrange the order of the symbols – for example, telling Sarah to give the apple to Peony, another chimpanzee. When that happened, Sarah would often refuse, or reorder the symbols to indicate that the apple should be given to her not Peony, suggesting that she understood that the symbols placed in a different order had different meanings. It looked as though Sarah understood grammar. As Sarah's comprehension developed, she was able to respond to more complicated sentences such as "Sarah banana blue pail insert." When presented with

---

[23] Hess 2008.   [24] Terrace, et al. 1979.

both bananas and apples, red and blue pails, and red and blue dishes, Sarah would accurately place the correct fruit in the correct colored pail or dish the majority of the time.

As remarkable as Sarah's comprehension of this symbolic, representational form of communication was, she did not use it to initiate discussions or to construct sentences, as human language users do. The researchers who worked with Sarah originally, David and Ann Premack, showed that chimpanzees were not just responding to cues from researchers, as skeptics believed. But while Sarah was able to use a representational system, the Premacks concluded that the most advanced representation, the sentence, was "far beyond the capacity of the chimpanzee."[25] So, it is the ability to construct sentences, and not merely use language, that makes humans unique.

Sue Savage-Rumbaugh, who works with bonobos, has been critical of the bar-raising dialectic of these debates, suggesting, as I do, that they are misguided attempts by those who cling to the idea of an insurmountable divide between humans and other animals to establish human exceptionalism – even in the face of clear evidence establishing continuities between human skills and the skills used by some non-humans. Every time an ape is able to do something characteristic of human language usage, skeptics either deny it actually happened or minimize the significance of that activity. Savage-Rumbaugh took on the challenge of sentence comprehension by asking Kanzi, the bonobo she worked with, to do very odd things. Like Sarah, Kanzi would readily put bananas in blue pails or apples in green dishes when asked, but now Savage-Rumbaugh was asking Kanzi to put pails on bananas, pine needles in the refrigerator, and soap on a ball. Kanzi did remarkably well, given that he was asked to do things he had never seen done before and that seem nonsensical, probably even to him. Kanzi's younger sister, Panbanisha, did even better.[26]

Still, some skeptics remained unconvinced that other animals were, in fact, comprehending language. Steven Pinker, a cognitive scientist who studies language acquisition in children, for example, thinks what Kanzi and others are engaged in is mere associative learning. He thinks the apes have undergone a complex form of training, and as a result, they have learned how to press the right buttons or do the right behaviors in order to get the hairless apes who train them to cough up M&M's, bananas, and other desirable tidbits of food.

[25] Premack & Premack 1984: 123.   [26] Savage-Rumbaugh, et al. 1998.

While the apes had to be taught to use language, just as we are taught to use language, their ability to teach each other, to generate words they haven't been taught by combining those they know, and to comprehend novel grammatical structures goes beyond simple training. Of course, those who believe the capacity for language is innate in humans, like linguist Noam Chomsky, will never be convinced. By definition, no other animals can use language, because it is wired into the human brain. As Chomsky says, "attempting to teach linguistic skills to animals is irrational – like trying to teach people to flap their arms and fly."[27]

Defining humans as unique in their capacity to use human language is akin to saying only humans have human intelligence. But we don't want to define away the possibility that the capacities or skills that make up human intelligence might be shared by others. If we approach other animals as if they are so different from us that we cannot imagine them behaving in fascinatingly familiar ways, we may overlook what they are doing and fail to ask the right questions about the cognitive bases for their behaviors. If we expect that they don't have the requisite capacities, then we might miss certain complex behaviors or interpret those behaviors in deflationary ways. Our commitment to human uniqueness may bias our observations and even the way that empirical research is conducted. This is precisely what happened when a new capacity was proposed that many thought was surely unique to humans – the capacity to ascribe mental states to others.

Theory of mind

Being able to understand that another being feels, sees, and thinks, and to get a sense of what those emotions, perceptions, and thoughts might be, requires a fairly complex set of cognitive skills. Someone who has a theory of mind (ToM), as this complex set of cognitive skills is called, has to understand, at a minimum, that they are individuals who are distinct from the other; that the other has experiences, perceptions, and thoughts; and that those may be different from one's own. Humans above the age of four are generally able to think about what others might be thinking. Most human teenagers seem to be obsessed with thinking about what others think. But does this complex cognitive capacity make humans unique?

---

[27] Cited in Johnson 1995: C10. See also, Chomsky 1980 and Lloyd 2004.

The question of another animal possibly possessing the cognitive capacity to recognize others as cognitive beings was first posed by Guy Woodruff and David Premack in their 1978 article "Does the Chimpanzee Have a Theory of Mind?" According to them, to have a ToM, a being "imputes mental states to himself and to others (either to conspecifics or to other species as well)." Woodruff and Premack suggested that the types of mental states that would be attributed to others might include "purpose, intention, beliefs, thinking, knowledge, pretending, liking, and doubt."[28] In order to answer their question, Woodruff and Premack modified Wolfgang Köhler's "insight" experiments with chimpanzees. While directing the Anthropoid Station in Tenerife, Köhler presented chimpanzees with the problem of obtaining bananas hanging just out of reach in their enclosure. They had bamboo poles and tools nearby, and, according to Köhler, the chimpanzees would suddenly arrive at the correct combination of actions needed to reach the bananas, leading him to speculate that the chimpanzees had a sudden insight allowing them to perceive the solution to the problem. In Woodruff and Premack's experiments, rather than presenting a problem for Sarah to solve, they videotaped humans trying to solve problems, like how to obtain the out-of-reach bananas with poles and boxes. Woodruff and Premack showed the videotapes to Sarah to determine whether she would be able to recognize that the human was trying to solve a problem by indicating or predicting how the human would solve each problem.

Four thirty-second videotapes were made of a human actor in a cage trying to obtain bananas that were inaccessible. In addition to the videos, still photographs were taken of the human actor engaged in a behavior constituting the solution to the problems. Sarah was shown each video, until the last five seconds, at which point the video was put on hold. Sarah was then shown two photographs, only one of which represented a solution to the problem. The experimenter left the room, and Sarah selected one of the two photographs by placing her selection in a designated location. Sarah made the correct selection in twenty-one of twenty-four trials. So, it looked as though Sarah understood that the human actor was attempting to achieve a particular goal, understood that he faced a problem that he wanted to overcome, and was able to determine what would allow the actor to overcome the problem to reach his goal. To be able to do that, Sarah would have to attribute "at least

---

[28] Woodruff and Premack 1978: 518.

two states of mind to the human actor, namely, intention or purpose on the one hand, and knowledge or belief on the other."[29]

However, because there were a number of possible alternative explanations to the theory of mind hypothesis – namely, that Sarah's behavior could be explained through association learning or empathy, Woodruff and Premack expanded Sarah's tests in an attempt to eliminate the possibility that Sarah was either generalizing old situations to predict new ones (rather than attributing mental states) or that she was simply putting herself in the place of the human actor (simulating rather than reasoning).

To control for association learning, Sarah was shown four novel videotaped scenarios requiring her, again, to choose the photograph representing the solution to the problem in the video. Sarah performed significantly better than chance. To control for empathy, the actors in the videos were now a former acquaintance of Sarah's to whom she showed no affection and, alternatively, Sarah's favorite caregiver. Sarah selected the right responses to solve the problem for the actor she liked and selected the wrong responses, failing to solve the problem, for the actor she didn't care for at a highly significant rate. This meant that she wasn't putting herself into the position of the human but, instead, could recognize distinct humans, solving the problem for the human she liked and not solving the problem for the human she didn't.[30]

From this series of tests, Woodruff and Premack concluded that future research would show that chimpanzees can correctly attribute wants, intentions, and purposes to others. It appeared that some animals, other than humans, had a theory of mind, only it wasn't as sophisticated as human theory of mind. However, as was the case with tool use and language use, some people denied that this work defeated human exceptionalism. In response, specifically focused experiments were conducted to determine whether chimpanzees could pass what are called "non-verbal false belief tests," often used with human children before they can speak. A test was designed to determine whether chimpanzees understood that seeing meant knowing. Two humans would stand outside an enclosure with a desirable food item. One of the

---

[29] Ibid.: 515.

[30] I have known Sarah for many years (although not when she was performing these particular tests) and the observation about helping someone she likes and not helping someone she doesn't like sounds just like Sarah to me.

humans would not be able to see the chimpanzee. (Her eyes might be covered; she would have a bucket over her head; or she would be looking away.) The other human would be looking right at the chimpanzee. If the chimpanzee went to the human that could see him and asked for food, rather than going to the human who could not see him to ask for food, researchers could conclude that the chimpanzees understood that seeing was an important part of the way individuals formed mental states. Chimpanzees approached the humans randomly in this set of experiments.[31] None of this work supported the original conclusion that chimpanzees could attribute wants, intentions, beliefs, or purposes to themselves or others. Indeed, quite the opposite was being claimed. For example, in her 1998 article, Cecilia Heyes suggested that "there is still no convincing evidence of theory of mind in primates. We should stop asking Premack & Woodruff's question."[32]

There are a number of reasons why convincing evidence that chimpanzees had a theory of mind was lacking. One was that the standards for what would count as evidence kept changing as the meaning of ToM kept changing. For example, Heyes writes, "an animal with a theory of mind believes that mental states play a causal role in generating behavior and infers the presence of mental states in others by observing their appearance and behavior under various circumstances."[33] To have a theory of mind under this definition is not just to make attributions of mental states to others in predicting their behavior but also to have a view about how those mental states causally affect the behavior. This involves having a concept of causation. Like the tool use and language use debates, it looked like the bar was getting higher for what it meant to have a theory of mind.

Then Brian Hare and his colleagues noticed that chimpanzees did seem to understand something about the visual perception of other chimpanzees.[34] Hare created an experiment in which a subordinate chimpanzee and a dominant chimpanzee were put in competition over food, and showed that the subordinate would systematically approach the food the dominant could not see and avoid the food the dominant could see.[35] In a variation on this theme, a subordinate watched food being hidden that the dominant could only sometimes see, depending on whether or not the dominant chimpanzee's door was open or closed during the time of hiding. When the dominant was released,

---

[31] Povinelli, et al. 1996.   [32] Heyes 1998: 102.   [33] Ibid.
[34] Hare, et al. 2000.   [35] Hare & Tomasello 2001.

the subordinate would only approach the food that the dominant had not seen being hidden, even though the dominant could see it now. After a series of experiments, the researchers claimed, "We therefore believe that these studies show what they seem to show, namely that chimpanzees actually know something about the content of what others see and, at least in some situations, how this governs their behavior."[36] They concluded, "At issue is no less than the nature of human cognitive uniqueness. We now believe that our own and others' previous hypotheses to the effect that chimpanzees do not understand any psychological states at all were simply too sweeping."[37] The researchers attribute the chimpanzee's success in demonstrating an understanding of another's psychological state to the ecological relevancy of the experiment. Food competition, they suggest, rather than begging for food from a human, is a more species-typical behavior and is, therefore, more likely to be accompanied by complex social cognitive abilities.

Although there is still some debate about what exactly these ecologically relevant changes mean in terms of whether chimpanzees have a theory of mind, it is interesting to recognize that chimpanzees may be more interested in solving problems that appear "natural" to them. When researchers stepped back and observed what the chimpanzees tended to do when interacting among themselves, and then designed the experiments based on those observations, the results were markedly different than those that emerged when the experimental paradigm was designed as if chimpanzees were socially and behaviorally like human children. What counts as a "natural" problem, particularly for individuals who have spent their entire lives in captivity, is itself an interesting question we will explore in the next chapter. The acknowledgment that we may learn more when we look at other animals behaving in ways that are species-typical is an important insight that will certainly help us to understand their cognitive processes. Their way of seeing us and their worlds may turn out to be quite different than the way we see them and imagine they see our world.

Ethical engagement

Some have argued that what makes humans unique is our ability to engage in ethical behavior. Surely, no other animals can be said to act morally. Yet, it

---

[36] Tomasello, et al. 2003: 155.   [37] Ibid.: 156.

does seem that when the dolphins mentioned at the beginning of this chapter were protecting the New Zealand swimmers from the great white shark they were engaging in something like ethical behavior. In order to determine whether or not it makes sense to think of dolphins and other animals as ethical beings, or whether humans are the lone residents of an ethical universe, we need to have a working definition of morality, keeping in mind that there have been long-standing and unresolved religious, philosophical, and scientific debates about the definition and domain of morality. If morality requires scrutinizing one's reasons for acting and deciding whether those reasons would justify that particular action – which seems to require language and, possibly, a theory of mind – then we are back to the debates just reviewed. For some philosophers in the Kantian tradition, this is what morality consists of – being able to formulate a principle of action, to reflect on that principle, and, ultimately, to determine whether it can be willed to be a universal law. And if that is what it means to be ethical, then in all likelihood no other animals are ethical, and it may turn out that some humans aren't either. (We'll discuss that possibility further in the next chapter.) However, if we think of morality as involving other-regarding concerns and behaviors, then it may well be that other animals could be considered moral. Protecting the sick or weak (sometimes referred to as altruistic behavior), cooperation, acting empathetically, and following norms all look like moral behaviors and animals seem to engage in behaviors that can be described in these ways.

In Bossou in West Africa, chimpanzees are occasionally observed crossing roads that intersect with their territories. One of the roads is busy with traffic; the other is mostly a pedestrian route; and both are dangerous to the chimpanzees. On videotaped recordings of chimpanzee behavior at the crossings, researchers observed that adult males took up forward and rear positions, with adult females and young occupying the more protected middle positions. The position of the dominant and bolder individuals, in particular the alpha male, changed depending on both the degree of risk and number of adult males present. Researchers suggested that cooperative action in the higher-risk situation was probably aimed at maximizing group protection.[38] This sort of risk-taking for the sake of others is often observed in male patrols of territorial boundaries in other parts of Africa. In these instances, a bold male, who may or may not be the alpha of the group, together with others

[38] Hockings, et al. 2006.

with whom he has an alliance, begins a patrol with the goal of obtaining potential food rewards, as well as of protecting the group from neighboring threats.[39]

Frans de Waal and Sarah Brosnan conducted experiments to analyze cooperative food-sharing behavior among chimpanzees and capuchin monkeys in captivity. They found that adults were more likely to share food with individuals who had groomed them earlier in the day. Grooming involves one individual using his or her hands to look through another chimpanzee's coat, picking out nits, inspecting for injuries, but mostly the behavior seems to provide enjoyment for the one being groomed and the one grooming. De Waal and Brosnan suggested that their results could be explained in two ways: the "good-mood hypothesis," in which individuals who have received grooming are in a benevolent mood and respond by sharing with all individuals, or the "exchange hypothesis," in which the individual who has been groomed responds by sharing food only with the groomer. The data indicated that the sharing was specific to the previous groomer. The chimpanzees remembered who had performed a service (grooming) and responded to that individual by sharing food. De Waal and Brosnan also observed that grooming between individuals who rarely did so was found to have a greater effect on sharing than grooming between partners who commonly groomed each other. Among partnerships in which little grooming was usually exchanged, there was a more pronounced effect of previous grooming on subsequent food sharing. They suggest that being groomed by an individual who doesn't usually groom might be more noticeable and, thus, warrant greater response in the form of food sharing, or it could be what they call "calculated reciprocity." They write: "not only do the chimpanzees regulate their food sharing based on previous grooming, but they recognize unusual effort and reward accordingly."[40] In a different set of studies, de Waal and his collaborators described reconciliation behaviors in which a high-ranking female will work to help two male chimpanzees "make up" after an altercation. This kind of behavior, in which the female first attends to the "winner," then reassures the "loser" and encourages him to follow her to a grooming session with the winner, has no obvious or immediate benefit for the female, but does impact social harmony. Once the males begin grooming each other, she will usually leave them alone.[41]

[39] Muller & Mitani 2005.   [40] Brosnan & de Waal 2002: 141.   [41] de Waal 2000.

Recently, Christopher Boesch and his colleagues reported eighteen cases of adoption of orphaned chimpanzees in the Tai forest of Côte d'Ivoire. They describe the adoption of the youngsters, and the extended care it requires, as altruistic behavior. Interestingly, half of the adoptions were done by males, only one of whom proved to be the father. From this fascinating set of observations the researchers concluded that "under the appropriate socio-ecologic conditions, chimpanzees do care for the welfare of other unrelated group members."[42]

And it is not just chimpanzees that engage in altruistic, cooperative, peacemaking, other-regarding behaviors. Marc Bekoff, an ethologist who studies canid play behavior and has written widely on animal behavior, recounts numerous examples of moral behaviors in other animals:

A teenage female elephant nursing an injured leg is knocked over by a rambunctious hormone-laden teenage male. An older female sees this happen, chases the male away, and goes back to the younger female and touches her sore leg with her trunk... A rat in a cage refuses to push a lever for food when it sees that another rat receives an electric shock as a result. A male Diana monkey who learned to insert a token into a slot to obtain food helps a female who can't get the hang of the trick, inserting the token for her and allowing her to eat the food reward. A female fruit-eating bat helps an unrelated female give birth by showing her how to hang in the proper way... A large male dog wants to play with a younger and more submissive male. The big male invites his younger partner to play and when they play, the big dog restrains himself and bites his younger companion gently and allows him to bite gently in return. Do these examples show that animals display moral behavior, that they can be compassionate, empathic, altruistic, and fair? Yes they do. Animals not only have a sense of justice, but also a sense of empathy, forgiveness, trust, reciprocity, and much more as well.[43]

Humans are much more sophisticated at large-scale cooperation, and, of course, only humans engage in moral theorizing. But we shouldn't forget that we are also capable of engaging in tremendously evil acts. As one reporter put it: "We're a species that is capable of almost dumbfounding kindness... And at the same time... we've visited untold horrors on ourselves... [think of] all of the crimes committed by the highest, wisest, most principled species

---

[42] Boesch, et al. 2010.   [43] Bekoff 2009: 1. See also Bekoff & Pierce 2009.

the planet has produced. That we're also the lowest, cruelest, most blood-drenched species is our shame – and our paradox."[44]

While there are obvious differences between humans and other animals, these differences are, as Darwin noted, ones "of degree and not of kind."[45] I have discussed only a small amount of the fascinating work on animal cognition suggesting that other animals may have some of the cognitive skills that were once thought to be unique to humans. These capacities have been observed in less elaborate form in other animals, and, usually, the more complex cognitive capacities tend to be exhibited in our closest living animal relatives, the great apes, but not always. Because human behavior and cognition share deep evolutionary roots with the behavior and cognition of other animals, approaches that try to find sharp behavioral or cognitive boundaries between humans and other animals will have to fill significant explanatory gaps.

What we can take away from this discussion is that the empirical search for a capacity or set of capacities that distinguishes humans from all other animals has lead to rich and provocative understandings of other animals and of ourselves, yet it has not provided a definitive conclusion about what is unique to all humans. Whether the study of other animals, particularly in their natural settings, is motivated by an interest in finding unique differences or in studying evolutionary continuities, what we have learned can usefully inform our attitudes and our behavior toward other animals. This is a welcome result from investigations that, at times, generated somewhat fruitless debates. And even though the empirical task of finding the capacity that makes humans unique has not yet led to definitive conclusions, one conclusion we certainly cannot draw is that humans and other animals are indistinguishable. All animals are different one from the other, as members of biological groups and as individuals. Chimpanzees are closer to humans genetically and evolutionarily than either is to another great ape, the gorilla. All great apes are markedly different from ungulates, carnivores quite distinct from herbivores, monotremes very unlike cats. Some animals spend their lives with their families, while others leave as soon as they are able. Some animals form lifelong pair-bonds; others are promiscuous. Humans have these variations, too. Given the tremendous variety of animal shapes, sizes, social structures, behaviors, and habitats, creating a human–animal divide really is

[44] Kluger 2007.   [45] Darwin 1888: 193.

a peculiar way to categorize organisms. Yet, marking difference in this way serves multiple purposes and is not necessarily meant to be biologically, functionally, or even conceptually neat. The divide in many ways supports, and perhaps results from, human exceptionalism that requires conceptualizing animals as others, particularly others of lesser worth.

Does difference matter morally?

Though there are many ways that humans are different from other animals, the truly problematic feature of human exceptionalism is its second implicit claim: the normative claim that elevates humans above other animals. By "normative," I mean evaluative – having to do with right and wrong, good and bad, valuable or worthless. "Normative" has a more popular meaning alluding to social expectations and what society views as "normal." The social norms in most parts of the world, though often very different, are similar in one respect – they tend toward human exceptionalism. People are expected to value humans above other animals. That is what is "normative" in the popular sense. In fact, people who focus too much on animals, or who treat their companion animals as children, for example, are often thought to be pretty weird, not quite "normal." I am not concerned here with this sense of normative – that is, what people think makes humans unique or what society judges to be uniquely valuable in humans. Rather I am interested in why, from a more abstract philosophical perspective, having some capacity makes the possessor better or worthy of more ethical concern than someone who doesn't have that capacity. The normative in this sense has to do with the ethical weight we attach to some capacity that makes humans exceptional. Suppose I have a really good friend who is a math wiz; he is exceptionally good at it. He has a capacity that I don't have. I'm not bad at math; I just have to work very hard at it. Neither of us thinks that because he finds math easy and I find it hard that he is better than me from an ethical perspective. His skill with math just makes him the better choice if there is a calculus problem in need of solution. That he is really good at math doesn't give him more rights, or more of a claim to ethical attention from others. We have equal rights and equal claims to moral attention. There are certain traits or capacities – being good at math, tall, blonde, bilingual (the list could go on) – that simply do not make a difference from an ethical point of view. They are irrelevant to thinking about what humans deserve or the way in which our claims to respect or equal treatment are addressed.

So which traits or capacities are relevant from an ethical point of view? This is another way of asking the question we are concerned with in this section. Let us suppose for the sake of argument that there is some empirically identifiable behavior, or capacity X, that is unique to human beings. Suppose it is the case that only humans use sophisticated toolkits or language with a generative grammar or have the capacity to attribute mental states to others. Why are those capacities what makes an individual deserving of moral attention? Why do these differences make a moral difference?

Those who advocate human exceptionalism as an ethical stance must provide answers to these questions. In virtue of what do all and only humans matter morally? Let's suppose the answer is that all, and only, humans matter because we use language. We would now want to ask *why* this is the capacity that matters. There are a number of answers that could be given. Those who use language can articulate their needs and interests and make direct claims on others who might otherwise neglect those needs or violate those interests. If someone is encroaching on me or acting in a way I deem wrong or harmful, I can say so. (Of course, whether or not I'm heard or understood is another matter.) I can use language to express my disapproval or to demand recognition. I can protest certain types of unethical actions with language. Since language is required to develop and convey ethical norms and expectations, and language is the means by which we teach those norms and correct violations, perhaps it is the capacity that indicates that humans are uniquely deserving of moral concern.

These are important reasons that speak in favor of considering language-users within the sphere of moral concern, but the class of language-users is not identical to the class of humans. Not all humans have this capacity, so human exceptionalism may not actually apply to all humans. If the boundary for inclusion in the class of morally considerable beings is drawn around all, and only, language-users, then humans who do not use language will not be the subjects of moral concern. They will be outside of the sphere. If they are outside the sphere delineating to whom ethical consideration is warranted, then ethical issues would not directly arise in our interactions with and treatment of them. They would only matter indirectly, as long as those who matter directly had an interest in them. If they were not of concern to language-users, the only individuals that matter directly on this account, then non-linguistic humans could be used, enslaved, even killed, and that would not be ethically wrong.

This is a frightening conclusion to draw. Humans who don't use language still have interests and needs that we generally think should be of moral concern. When we think about acts of ethical heroism – running up the stairs as a skyscraper is collapsing to try to save people, jumping into a chimpanzee enclosure to try to save a chimp who has fallen into the moat and is drowning, running into a burning building to rescue a family rendered unconscious due to smoke inhalation – there often isn't communication in those instances, either because those in need are unconscious, don't possess developed language abilities, or there just isn't time to talk. And it isn't the fact that they could use language that makes saving them right and important. We don't thank the firefighter for saving the family of language-users. Risking one's own well-being to protect the well-being of another is seldom based on a determination of whether or not the individual is a language-user. We don't generally think of language use as a necessary condition for moral consideration in the case of humans.

It might be argued that we don't need to have conversations with humans in danger to know that they are in trouble. If the circumstances were different, they would use language to tell us that they would like their interests and needs protected. Indeed, language is what allows us to organize and develop emergency response teams who can go out and successfully do the right thing in times of trouble.

While this is all true, and our ability to communicate through language is a valuable capacity, being able to communicate through language isn't tied to the ability to experience undesirable states. Language helps us communicate our desire not to be in such states, but it is being in such a state, not our ability to express it, that matters morally. It isn't only linguistic beings who may experience distress. And we know this because non-linguistic beings – human infants, humans with particular sorts of cognitive deficits, and other animals – are capable of expressing their interests and needs without language. They are certainly able to express distress, despair, and pain without language. Some non-linguistic animals are even capable of expressing disapproval; when an individual in their social group acts in ways that are inappropriate, others in the group will punish the one who is misbehaving. Given that interests and needs can be communicated both through language as well as through other non-verbal forms of communication and practices, the capacity to use language does not appear to be necessary for inclusion in the sphere of moral concern.

The ability to use tools, possession of a theory of mind, planning ahead, having a sense of humor, pointing to get someone's attention, and engaging in cooperation, all require cognitive skills, skills that are characteristic of normal adult human beings. But they are not capacities that all humans have, and, as we've seen, it may very well be that some other animals do have these capacities, often in less sophisticated forms. Not all humans have the exact same set of unique cognitive capacities, and if human exceptionalism is meant to help us see why we should direct our moral attention to all and only humans, we will discover that the view is flawed, as many of the most vulnerable among us will be overlooked. Additionally, some other animals, maybe dolphins or great apes, have fairly impressive cognitive skills, and excluding them from moral attention simply because they are not human amounts to nothing more than morphological or species-based prejudice. Human exceptionalism, as an ethical position, is untenable.

Who is ethically considerable?

Since it seems that the boundary of moral concern cannot be drawn defensibly around humans based on some unique, ethically relevant capacity that all and only humans share, we cannot pay exclusive attention to the claims of only other humans. If we must pay attention to how our actions affect more than humans, though, how do we know to whom or to what to direct our moral attention? Who can make claims on us that demand a moral response and on what basis can such claims be made? Our lives are complicated, filled with all sorts of beings and things that are affected by our behavior both directly, through our immediate actions, and indirectly, through the choices and plans we make. Which of those beings and things ought we to consider from an ethical point of view?

Let's now turn to some suggestions about how to answer these questions. We will see that there are ways of answering these questions that extend the moral sphere far beyond humans and other animals, to include plants and all living beings, but in this section, we will primarily focus on why other animals should command our moral attention.

One way to approach the question of who matters morally is to imagine the following thought experiment. Suppose you have been abducted by aliens who, you fear, plan to do things to you that you would rather not have done. You decide you want to try to communicate with these aliens, and your hope is that they might respond to reason. A couple of aliens appear at the door of the enclosure where you are captive, and you decide to try to reason with your captors, encouraging them to return you to your life on Earth. What exactly would you say?

Imagine that you have figured out a way to communicate clearly with the aliens; your words don't sound like shrieks, hoots, or grunts to them. You might express your desire not to be held captive, that being held against your will is wrong, and that it prevents you from doing not just the things you want to be doing at home, but the things you are supposed to be doing. These aliens are frustrating your desires and preventing you from fulfilling your obligations to others. You might explain that you are a rational and sensitive individual who has immediate desires and long-term plans that you hope to satisfy. You don't think you should be treated as a means to some alien ends. You might try to bargain with them, telling them you will do something for them if they do something for you. You have relationships to others that you want to continue to pursue, and you would be willing to develop a relationship with them if they respect you. You value your freedom and your ability to make choices. You need to be with your friends, family, and others of your kind. If you are forced to stay with the aliens, you will become bored, frustrated, lonely, angry, and depressed. You may even die. Holding you captive, against your will, harms you in many, many ways.

Now let's imagine you are successful convincing the aliens, and after a few minutes you find yourself back in your own home. You persuaded the aliens that your interests and well-being are worthy of their moral attention. You probably would not have convinced them by saying you are human or a member of the species *Homo sapiens*. That was obvious when they abducted you, and it didn't matter to them at that point. What does matter, pointedly in this hypothetical case but importantly in our ordinary interactions, is that when there are values at stake, ethical agents are called to respond, and in our science fiction scenario it appears that the aliens thought of themselves as ethical agents and responded well.

If we turn this thought experiment around and put ourselves in the position of the aliens, or just see ourselves as conscientious ethical agents, and think of the animals we produce, fatten, and slaughter in industrial agriculture; those we experiment on in laboratories; those we hold captive in zoos, aquariums, and circuses; those we are destroying in their native habitats; and even those we have as pets, we can again imagine how they might respond to us if they were able to communicate with us in ways that didn't sound like shrieks, hoots, or grunts. As ethical agents, we want to make our way through the world taking the right sorts of actions, making the right sorts of choices, and doing good for, or at least preventing harm to, others. In thinking about other animals, then, we should consider whether our actions and our choices can do them good, promote their well-being, or, conversely, cause them harm.

In our hypothetical scenario, we identified a number of values that we wanted the aliens to recognize as providing them with reasons to act differently, to let us go. In the reversed situation, the values that are at stake will be different, depending on the animal that we might understand to be making the claim for our moral attention. Of course, in "making a claim" the animals will not actually be formulating sentences to express the values they want respected and promoted. They probably don't recognize such values as values. The challenge for us, as ethical agents who are responsive to values, is to try to identify what values are being threatened in their particular contexts, to try to make their claims on us understandable, and to act accordingly.

Living beings

Living a good life, in which individual well-being and flourishing is promoted, is not an uncommon goal, and it is one that most would like supported in an ethical world. Not only humans have this goal. The lives of all animals, humans and non-humans alike, can go better or worse for them. There are some things that are necessary for lives to go well, and discovering what those things are will provide a first step in recognizing what sort of values are at stake in a world where not everyone is in a position to lead a good life.

Having a life is certainly a fundamental value, and ending that life, other things being equal, would be a clear way of destroying something valuable. There are many philosophical difficulties here, and we will be exploring some of these in the chapters ahead. What is important for current purposes is to recognize that being alive is necessary for any other values to exist, and there is, thus, a prima facie reason for valuing life itself. From an ethical point of view there are vast differences between throwing away an inanimate object, like a chair, and killing a living being, like a cheetah. In the case of the inanimate object, there may be ethical questions that arise, for example, when considering the proper disposal of the chair. It would be a bad idea to throw the chair out of a window from a high-rise building onto a busy street below, but it wouldn't be bad for the chair, just the hapless passerby who might be hit by it. In the case of living beings, ending life has complex ethical implications, and it is usually bad for the one being killed. Consider the cheetah. We would want to know whether this individual is healthy and would be destined to live many more satisfying years. Destroying the cheetah under those conditions would be bad for the cheetah, as it would foreclose the possibility of having future valuable experiences. If the individual is terminally ill or gravely injured, or already at the end of his life and barely existing with a very low quality of life, then maybe killing him would not be so bad, but here, unlike the case of inanimate objects, there are distinct questions of values. For example, we may consider how the life of this individual affects the lives of others. Will killing the cheetah hurt his family? Will they be able to survive without him?

Plants, trees, and other parts of nature are also alive, and some theorists have argued that, insofar as life is valuable, all living things should be considered from an ethical point of view. Noted theologian Albert Schweitzer, for example, extolled a reverence for life and urged people to consider ending life only if it is absolutely necessary.

> Whenever I injure life of any sort, I must be quite clear whether it is
> necessary. Beyond the unavoidable, I must never go, not even with what
> seems insignificant. The farmer, who has mown down a thousand flowers in
> his meadow as fodder for his cows, must be careful on his way home not to
> strike off in wanton pastime the head of a single flower by the roadside, for he
> thereby commits a wrong against life without being under the pressure of
> necessity.[46]

In environmental ethics, biocentrists like Paul Taylor see all living things as "teleological centers of life" and, as such, deserving of ethical consideration.[47] Kenneth Goodpaster has also argued that all life matters from a moral point of view. Plants, he suggests, like animals, have interests, and those interests should be taken into account when making an ethical decision about life and death.[48]

---

[46] Schweitzer 1936.   [47] Taylor 1986.   [48] Goodpaster 1978.

Having interests

From an ethical point of view, the interests of all who have them should be taken into account. To favor someone's interests over another's, simply because you like, want to impress, or can relate to the first person, and dislike, don't care about, or can't relate to the second person, would be objectionably prejudicial. It is generally considered ethically wrong to engage in prejudicial considerations or considerations that cannot be justified through argumentation. It would seem to be prejudicial to ignore plant interests because they are just plants. But does this mean that we should consider the interests of a tree in not being chopped down as equivalent to the interests of a perfectly healthy college student in not being killed? In order to answer this question, we will need to be more precise about what we mean by "interests." There are two senses of interests. To say that A has an interest in X could mean that A is interested in X – that is, A likes X or is aiming at X. I could be interested in starting a sanctuary for primates no longer needed in biomedical research or the entertainment industry. I might spend hours thinking about where to locate the sanctuary. I might look for land, conduct research on ways to rehabilitate animals who have had traumatic lives, and visit existing sanctuaries. This sense of interest requires that I direct my intentions and actions in a particular way.

Another sense of the phrase "A has an interest in X" is that X will benefit A, that X is conducive to A's good. Perhaps I have a heart ailment that is made better by a particular vitamin supplement. Taking that supplement would be in my interests, but I needn't be interested in taking the supplement. A could be interested in X, but X may not be in A's interests; and X could be in A's interests, but A may not be at all interested in X. The two senses are distinct. Plants and trees may have interests in the second sense – that is, they are the sorts of things that can have their interests negatively affected, when they are chopped down, or lack water and light, but they will never be interested in that impact. Animals, on the other hand, are the sorts of beings that have both sorts of interests. Things can be against their interests, and they can intentionally direct their actions. Unlike plants, animals, both human and non-human, can express their interests as wants or desires that can be interpreted through their actions.

So, in addition to the value of life, all animals have interests in both senses and express those interests as wants or desires. Satisfying particular interests,

wants, and desires contributes to making a life a good life. Frustrating particular interests, wants, and desires diminishes well-being. Of course, there are
philosophical complications here, too. What if someone wants what is bad
for them, maybe they have distorted desires? Is there some objective way to
tell what interests, wants, and desires will be conducive to well-being, or does
it just depend on how the individual feels when his or her interests, wants,
and desires are satisfied? How do we know how another feels, particularly
if they are a different kind of animal? It will be worthwhile to explore this
debate about the nature and value of well-being a bit here as it will help us to
identify to what we should be ethically attending when we seek to promote
the interests of others.

Well-being

Some have argued that an individual has a high level of well-being if she has
attained some number of valuable things that can be represented on what has
been called an "objective list." So, for example, if a recent college graduate
has physical health and bodily integrity, is able to think freely and dream, has
meaningful loving relations with others with whom she can freely choose to
associate, pursues the good life and has achieved success, is able to live in a
healthy environment, and has time to laugh, play, relax, and enjoy herself,
then it could be said that she has a high level of well-being.[49] It would be hard
to argue that being healthy and having friendships, meaningful work, and
the like are not the sorts of things that are valuable and conducive to well-
being for humans. However, it might be suggested that, while these things
are generally conducive to our well-being, it is possible that the individual
who has them doesn't consider herself to be at a high level of well-being,
perhaps because these aren't the things that really matter to her. Perhaps,
what would constitute her well-being would be to live a purer, more pious
life, renouncing everything else in order to become more contemplative, and
she hasn't succeeded in that. Regardless of what can be observed from the
outside, if an individual's life does not contain the things that she herself finds
most valuable or important, then it would be a mistake to claim that she has

---

[49] This is a partial list that draws on Nussbaum 2000: 78–80. She extends her list to include
animals, as we will see in the next section.

well-being. Well-being cannot be judged externally; it must be experienced from the inside.

But if well-being is a mental state, which sorts of mental state or states constitute well-being? Hedonistic theories identify well-being with happiness or pleasure, where happiness and pleasure are desirable states of consciousness. But consider a possibility that the movie *The Matrix* makes vivid cinematically. In the movie, humans are used as batteries to sustain machines, and, in exchange, humans are given the illusion that they are having real lives, so that they have desirable states of consciousness.[50] The humans spend their entire lives in pods that maintain their vital functions. They don't move, they don't see, they don't interact and they have no real experiences. When a few of the humans living in this state become aware of it, they fight hard to leave the matrix to enter the "real world," and it seems obvious why. Being deceived into thinking that one is having pleasure, or that one has desirable consciousness, is not the same as having well-being. Well-being requires actual, not illusory, engagement with the world.

The possibility that one may be deceived into pleasurable mental states has led others to argue that well-being is more adequately captured by some version of "desire satisfaction theory." This sort of theory attempts to connect mental states – namely, desires – with the world through their satisfaction. Let's suppose that our recent college graduate desires the love of her family, a secure amount of wealth, and to be healthy, and that these desires are reasonable. Let's suppose further that she, in fact, has these things, yet she doubts that her loved ones love her, fears that she will lose all her money in a volatile stock market, and, even though she is healthy, worries that she has some catastrophic, incurable disease. According to a desire-satisfaction theory, only when she recognizes that her friends and family really do love her, that she has made wise investment decisions, and that she is in good health, will she have a high level of well-being. Her reasonable desires will be satisfied. Of course, it is also possible that she is suspicious and pessimistic by nature and no amount of evidence about how much she is actually loved, how secure her wealth is, and how healthy she is will change her view of her well-being. If this is the case, then the fact that her desires are satisfied will not change her subjective experience of her own level of well-being. She may have

---

[50] As a number of philosophers writing about *The Matrix* note, the movie represents a similar problem to Nozick's experience machine. See Nozick 1974 and Grau 2005.

uncorrectable misperceptions about her situation, believing that her desires have not been satisfied, and, as a result, a low level of well-being despite the fact that she has, indeed, satisfied her desires. So, the desire-satisfaction view, even though it ties well-being to the desires a person has, still doesn't capture well-being from the inside.

While it is hard to deny that an individual's sense of well-being must be experienced (sensed) from the inside, there are also objective conditions that must factor in to third-party determinations of well-being, factors that are of particular interest to us. This is especially important when we are trying to promote the well-being of those with whom we cannot directly communicate, such as other animals who cannot express in words what their subjective states are. What might these objective conditions be? All beings that have interests, wants, and desires are sentient, that is, they are capable of experiencing pleasures and pains. And all sentient beings require basic sorts of things in order to function at all.[51] The minimal conditions for such functioning – adequate nutrition and hydration, relative health and bodily integrity, shelter from the elements, a non-toxic living environment, freedom of movement, social engagement (for social beings), and freedom of expression in its various forms – seem non-controversial, and how these conditions are satisfied will vary depending on the type of animal being considered. An individual who is starving or sick, or who has been mutilated, poisoned, imprisoned, kept in solitary confinement, or silenced (either physically or psychologically) cannot be thought to have well-being. While the humans serving as batteries in *The Matrix* have their nutritional needs met, for example, and while they may believe they are happy and living meaningful lives, the minimal requirements for well-being are absent. Thus, they cannot be said to have well-being. This would also be true for individuals who are living in solitary confinement, even when they are fed, can walk around their cells, and are permitted to scream or sing or talk to themselves. If, against the odds,

---

[51] I am alluding here to Amartya Sen's functionings and capabilities account of well-being. According to Sen, "The well-being of a person can be seen in terms of the quality (the 'well-ness,' as it were) of the person's being. Living may be seen as consisting of a set of interrelated 'functionings,' consisting of beings and doings. . . . The relevant functionings can vary from such elementary things as being adequately nourished, being in good health, avoiding escapable morbidity and premature mortality, etc. to more complex achievements such as being happy, having self-respect, taking part in the life of the community and so on." Sen 1992: 39.

they are able to find some contentment or satisfaction in their thoughts, they nonetheless lack well-being. Other animals who are confined, or who have their lives controlled and bodies manipulated, also lack well-being, because they are denied the minimal requirements necessary for its achievement.

The avoidance of pain and the exercise of relative freedoms represent the basic interests of sentient beings. This sets a minimal limit on what ethical agents should attend to when they are seeking to promote well-being. So, to return us to our alien thought experiment: when you were attempting to reason with the aliens, you expressed the value of being sentient, of having interests and desires that were frustrated, of suffering physically and emotionally from being away from your home and family. These are values that we share with other sentient beings. You also expressed your value as an ethical agent: that you had obligations to others and autonomy that was being thwarted. It is not clear that other animals could make similar claims, and, as we'll see in the next chapter, there are some humans who can't either. If an individual is not autonomous in a certain sense, one in which freedom depends on the ability to reflect on actions and choices and make decisions about which of the actions one has reason to pursue, then denying that individual autonomy will not constitute a harm. But, as we will see in Chapter 5, there may be other ways of thinking about the meaning of autonomy. When we deny sentient beings their basic interests we cause them to suffer emotionally, physically, or both, and we are causing them harm. Other things being equal, from an ethical point of view, harming another is a source of concern. Of course, not all harms can be avoided. When interests conflict, as they often do in our world of limited resources, we need guidance on how to adjudicate these conflicts.

Attending to other animals

Other animals matter because, like us, their lives can go better or worse for them. They are sentient beings who have interests and well-beings. They can be harmed when their interests are thwarted and their wellness is undermined. In an ideal world, we would be able to live harmoniously with one another and with other animals, there would be no conflicts, and everyone would have their interests satisfied. We don't live in an ideal world. Insofar as we have to make choices about how to act ethically when interests conflict, having theoretical frameworks to guide our thinking and our actions will be most useful. Fortunately, philosophers have developed a variety of such frameworks to help us navigate difficult ethical terrain. These frameworks, usually referred to as normative ethical theories, tend to conflict with one another in principle, but very often lead to the same general conclusions about courses of action. They provide us with different types of reasons for acting in one way or another, but, on occasions, as we will see throughout this book, they can be used to build upon each other to support a more inclusive way of looking at our ethical obligations to other animals.

Utilitarianism

One of the strongest ethical theories to articulate how we ought to attend to other animals is utilitarianism. As a theory that is fundamentally concerned with maximizing pleasure and minimizing pain for all those affected by any given action, it is not hard to understand what motivated classical utilitarianism's founding father, Jeremy Bentham, to extend the theory to other animals. Bentham directly addressed the question we explored in the last section, but, for him, pleasure and pain are what matter. As he famously stated, it can't be "the number of the legs, the villosity of the skin, or the termination of the os sacrum ... What else is it that should trace the insuperable line? Is it the faculty of reason, or perhaps the faculty for discourse? ... The question is not, Can they reason? nor Can they talk? but Can they suffer?"[52] Utilitarians include all sentient beings, beings who can suffer, in their calculus to determine what actions are right and what actions are not. If a course of action will lead to more suffering than pleasure for all those who are affected by that action, then that action will be ethically impermissible. It doesn't matter if the suffering accrues to moles or men, or if the pleasure accrues to wombats or women. Once it is aggregated and compared, the course of action with the least suffering is the course of action ethically required.

Peter Singer, who is often thought of as the "father of the modern animal rights movement," argues for a more complex version of utilitarianism than Bentham's. His is a preference utilitarian view that applies to all beings who have preferences, and it actually has nothing to do with animal "rights" per se. Singer, like utilitarians before him, is concerned about promoting pleasure and minimizing suffering, not in establishing rights, particularly

[52] Bentham 1789: Ch. 17, n. 122.

rights that cannot be overridden by considerations of the greater good. For utilitarians, who seek to bring about the best consequences when all morally relevant interests are taken into account, rights can be violated if it would promote the most good. According to Singer, if a being suffers, that suffering must be taken into account along with the like suffering of others, and it doesn't matter what species the suffering being is. If it turns out, after all the interests in not suffering are taken into account, that the action that leads to the least overall suffering involves causing some suffering, maybe even some death, to goats or gibbons, for example, then that action will be justified. It is important to note that if less suffering overall would result by causing your grandmother to suffer, then that would be the right course of action, too. There is a difference, however, in Singer's view, between killing a goat and killing your grandmother, even if that killing is done painlessly. Although all like suffering is to be given equal consideration, painlessly killing a goat may be justified, whereas painlessly killing your grandmother may not be. This is because, arguably, your grandmother can explicitly formulate her preference for continued existence whereas the goat cannot. According to Singer, causing a being to suffer or violating that being's interests is wrong only when it fails to promote the greatest amount of interest satisfaction, all things considered. Put differently, if the way to promote greater happiness and interest satisfaction for humans as well as for other animals is by causing some beings, whether human or not, to suffer, then causing that necessary suffering is justified. Causing unnecessary suffering to humans or other animals is not, other things being equal, justified. For Singer, causing any animal to suffer is a matter of ethical concern and something to be avoided, particularly if there are different options available. However, if the only course of action that will promote the most good for humans and other animals involves some suffering, then that course of action would be the ethical course of action.

Singer's view, like other utilitarian views, is egalitarian in that it requires that we take like interests into account equally, no matter who has those interests. But equal consideration does not mean identical treatment. A horse's interest in having a good meal and your brother's interest in having a good meal are equal interests, and if there were a way to satisfy those interests, then that would promote the greatest happiness. However, the way those interests are satisfied will be very different. Your brother may "eat like a horse," but, in reality, would probably not be very happy with a horse's meal, and a horse probably would eat very little of the meal your brother typically eats.

Giving equal consideration to equal interests will often require following very different courses of action in order to satisfy those interests.

As we'll see in Chapter 4, one of the most controversial issues for utilitarians like Singer is the use of other animals in invasive biomedical research. Much of the justification for conducting this sort of research on other animals, even painful research, is utilitarian. Many of those who experiment on other animals believe that the pain and distress that is caused to rats and rabbits in research laboratories is much less than it would be if the research were performed on human beings. And they claim that the hoped-for benefits promise to outweigh the pain, suffering, and death experienced by animal subjects in the experiments.

Rights views

Animal rights proponents, like philosopher Tom Regan, take exception to such utilitarian views. To allow for the use of animals flagrantly treats all animals (humans and other animals) as means to some end, rather than treating every individual with the respect they are due. For Regan, we shouldn't look at each case and try to determine, based on the pleasure, pain, frustration, satisfaction, etc., whether it is right or wrong.

> The forlornness of the veal calf is pathetic, heart wrenching; the pulsing pain of the chimp with electrodes planted deep in her brain is repulsive; the slow, tortuous death of the raccoon caught in the leg-hold trap is agonizing. But what is wrong isn't the pain, isn't the suffering, isn't the deprivation. The fundamental wrong is the system that allows us to view animals as *our resources*, here for *us*.[53]

According to Regan, all normal adult humans and other animals are what he calls "subjects of a life" who have inherent worth and are due respect. Utilitarians, because they are focused on considerations of the greater good, reduce individuals to their usefulness to something bigger than them, making them only instrumentally worthy. As it is sometimes put, utilitarians view humans and other animals as mere containers of value, not beings who are valuable in themselves. Utilitarians cannot respect the distinct intrinsic value of individual lives. In order to protect that value, Regan argues we must

[53] Regan 1985: 13–26.

recognize all subjects of a life as having rights. Subjects of a life are beings with relatively complex mental lives that include perceptions, desires, beliefs, memories, intentions, and at least a minimal sense of the future. Precisely who is a subject of a life is open to some debate. (For example, do octopuses have this sort of mental life? What about bats?) But the basic idea is that the lives of these individuals matter to them, and this is what grounds their worth and is why they have rights.

The rights view holds that treating subjects of a life as resources is an injustice that must be remedied, not reformed. As Regan writes, "to reform injustice is to prolong injustice."[54] The unjust exploitation of other animals for food, in scientific research, or for entertainment must be abolished. The rights position is often thought to be an absolutist position, one that opposes appeals to improving the well-being of animals while ignoring the larger structures of exploitation in which they exist. In Chapter 7 we'll explore how this view informs social activism.

Feminist ethics

Feminist scholars have raised concerns about the adequacy of both utilitarianism and the rights view as the basis for guiding our action and attention toward other animals. The alternative theory, called a feminist ethic of care by Josephine Donovan and Carol Adams, expresses a variety of insightful criticisms of the dominant ethical views.[55] While there are a number of variations within the feminist care tradition, most proponents reject the detached calculations of utilitarianism and the oversimplification and absolutism of the rights-based approach. Instead, feminist care ethics views other animals as beings with whom we are in relationships, and it is within these complex relationships that animals command our ethical attention. Some of these relationships will be relationships of dependency, as with our companion animals; others will be relationships of power, as when animals have their lives and, ultimately, deaths controlled by economic and political interests. Attention to both the personal and the political forces that shape our relations is central to guiding our actions, as is caring and respectful consideration of the other. Of course, attention to the individual animals' experiences is also central. In order to respond ethically to the needs and interests of other

---

[54] www.cultureandanimals.org/pop1.html.   [55] See Donovan & Adams 2007.

animals, ethical agents need to develop empathetic skills allowing them to understand the experiences of another, as well as to situate those experiences in a larger social, political, and economic context.[56] With other animals, we are most often at some distance from their pain, distress, fear, confusion, and suffering. Developing empathy with and awareness of the way others experience the world is, thus, one of the ethical obligations that arises from a feminist ethic of care. Without such awareness, we cannot know what another animal needs or wants, what he may be nervous about, or when he is annoyed or content, and, thus, we cannot accurately respond until we develop it. Because non-humans cannot explicitly tell us what is in their interests, we must develop skills to understand them across our differences.

Capabilities approach

One way we might do that is to identify the interests that other animals have that, when fulfilled, lead to their flourishing. Martha Nussbaum has generated a list in her work that extends the capabilities approach that she and Amartya Sen developed for humans to non-human animals.[57] This list is an objective list of the sort that I discussed in the previous section, and, thus, it has some of the drawbacks that objective theories of well-being have – namely, that an individual may have all the things on the list but still not feel like they have well-being. Nonetheless, the account may prove less problematic in the case of non-human animals than in humans, precisely because it provides a rough guideline for the promotion of individual flourishing without relying on the subjective experiences of other animals which are often very difficult to ascertain fully.

According to Nussbaum, the standard views, particularly utilitarianism, do not take appropriate account of the value of activities that are required for a life of dignity. She writes:

> a good life, for an animal as for a human, has many different aspects: movement, affection, health, community, dignity, bodily integrity, as well as the avoidance of pain. Some valuable aspects of animal lives might not even lead to pain when withheld. Animals, like humans, often don't miss what they don't know, and it is hard to believe that animals cramped in small cages all their lives can dream of the free movement that is denied them. Nonetheless,

---

[56] See Cuomo & Gruen 1998 and Gruen 2009.   [57] Nussbaum 2006a.

it remains valuable as a part of their flourishing, and not just because its absence is fraught with pain. Even a comfortable immobility would be wrong for a horse, an elephant, or a gorilla. Those creatures characteristically live a life full of movement, space, and complex social interaction. To deprive them of those things is to give them a distorted and impoverished existence.[58]

Nussbaum sees her approach as an improvement over the standard approaches. Others have suggested that it is actually a helpful way to enhance our understanding of our utilitarian obligations or to flesh out what rights other animals might have. We needn't concern ourselves with whether the capabilities approach reduces to some other framework here. What is useful about this approach is the way that her list of "entitlements" can help us to focus more deeply on the values articulated in the previous section and to highlight in a concrete, rather than abstract, way how we might harm animals by violating their interests, and help them to flourish by promoting their capabilities.[59] As proponents of feminist care ethics would suggest, this list provides a useful guide for directing our empathetic attention.

Here are some of the capabilities or entitlements on Nussbaum's list (with my commentary):

1. *Life.* According to Nussbaum, "all animals are entitled to continue their lives, whether or not they have such a conscious interest." As I have already mentioned, all interests ultimately depend on life, so protecting an animal's life is, other things being equal, a central way to promote that individual's interests. Of course, if the life is full of unending pain, equivalent to a life not worth living, then extending that life may not be in the individual's interests. (This would apply to all animals, human and non-human.)

2. *Bodily Health.* This will vary by species, but all animals need proper nutrition and hydration and to be protected from cruelty and neglect.

3. *Bodily Integrity.* As Nussbaum writes, "animals have direct entitlements against violations of their bodily integrity by violence, abuse, and other forms of harmful treatment – whether or not the treatment in question is painful."

4. *Senses, Imagination, and Thought.* Animals under human control have every aspect of their lives determined for them. This is true of companion

[58] Nussbaum 2006b: B6–8.   [59] Nussbaum 2004: 314–17.

animals as much as it is of animals living in conditions of institutional use. Promoting this capability means allowing choices for animals in captivity, providing environmentally enriched enclosures, and supplying a variety of enrichment activities to allow the animals to engage in species-typical behaviors.

5. *Emotions*. Nussbaum suggests that "[Animals] are entitled to lives in which it is open to them to have attachments to others, to love and care for others, and not to have those attachments warped by enforced isolation or the deliberate infliction of fear." Recognizing animals as emotional beings will help us to address their emotional interests.

6. *Practical Reason*. While it may be difficult to extend the notion that non-humans have an interest in practical reason, the idea here seems to be that, insofar as other animals are capable of planning their activities, they ought to be provided with the opportunity to do so.

7. *Play*. According to Nussbaum, this is a centrally important capability for all sentient beings and reinforces the need for adequate space, freedom, and access to others of one's kind.

If satisfying these capabilities is an obligation that ethical agents have, then there will be some odd implications when it comes to human interactions with wild animals, as well as in certain cases with captive animals. For example, should we intervene in wild predation? If captive animals are traumatized by the presence of other members of their species and seem to prefer to be alone, should we force them to live with others? (This brings us back to the worry about objective v. subjective conceptions of good.) We will explore some of these issues in Chapter 6. Despite these challenges, the capabilities approach allows us to focus on the particular needs and abilities of other animals and provides us with a way to begin thinking about our specific obligations to them.

Virtue theory and continental approaches

There are two additional frameworks that address our ethical relationships with other animals. One has recently emerged from the continental philosophical tradition, the other from virtue ethics. Neither is action-guiding in the way that the standard rights-based frameworks and utilitarianism are. Like the feminist ethics approach, these traditions are critical of the type of argumentation utilized by the standard approaches, insofar as it tends to oversimplify and flatten our moral experiences and thus leaves too much out of the picture. Instead of focusing on protecting rights or preventing suffering, work about animals coming out of the continental and virtue ethics traditions urge us to reflect more deeply on our relations to animals and the way those relations shape our conceptions of ourselves and our agency.[60]

Continental philosophers pose philosophical questions differently than analytic philosophers. It could be said that continental philosophers tend toward bigger, more expansive inquiry, whereas analytic philosophers try to narrow and refine arguments. The standard ethical views about animals come out of the analytic tradition, and in order to maintain difference, some in the continental vein have eschewed talk about "ethics" altogether. Yet, when it comes to "the question of the animal," turning away from ethics is difficult. Jacques Derrida took the challenge face on at the end of his life by exploring the complex problems that "the animal" poses. He suggested that the look of an animal calls into question not only our certainty about the world but our very humanity. Standing naked before his cat, Derrida reflects on the subject that the cat as Other brings into focus – the vulnerable human, limited in his understanding of the world by language but connected to the Other through the finitude of the body. Cora Diamond, who similarly rejects analytic philosophical arguments about our ethical interactions with other animals, suggests that we need, instead, to see other animals as members of our communities who pull on us. It is in virtue of this pull that we will come to acknowledge what is ethically wrong with cruelty, for example.[61] When we confront other animals as fellow creatures, we recognize the ways that we share a common life, and this recognition allows us to see them as they are and us as we are.

Relatedly, some virtue theorists have recently argued that using other animals is wrong, not because it is a violation of the animal's rights or because, on balance, such an act creates more suffering than other acts. Rather, in using them in ways that are harmful or destructive to them, we display moral failings that reflect poorly on us as ethical agents. The traits of character we might associate with mature members of the moral community – kindness, sensitivity, compassion, generosity, and responsiveness – are what should

---

[60] Thanks to Kari Weil for insightful conversations about these approaches.
[61] Diamond 2001 and Clarke 1977.

be displayed in our dealings with all animals, human and non-human. As Rosalind Hursthouse recognized after having been exposed to alternative ways of seeing animals:

> I began to see [my attitudes] that related to my conception of flesh-foods as unnecessary, greedy, self-indulgent, childish, my attitude to shopping and cooking in order to produce lavish dinner parties as parochial, gross, even dissolute. I saw my interest and delight in nature programmes about the lives of animals on television and my enjoyment of meat as side by side at odds with one another ... Without thinking animals had rights, I began to see both the wild ones and the ones we usually eat as having lives of their own, which they should be left to enjoy. And so I changed. My perception of the moral landscape and where I and the other animals were situated in it shifted.[62]

The latter two types of approaches to animal ethics help us to rethink our relationships with other animals and to begin to recognize that our very conceptions of our selves is ultimately tied to our thinking and actions toward them. These approaches, and some feminist approaches as well, provide a means, through reflection, sensitivity, compassion, and empathy, to internalize the moral demands that animals' claims make on us. The standard views provide us with external guidance for action, often in abstract or detached ways. Thinking about all of the frameworks together can provide what philosophers call both "internal and external reasons" for treating animals ethically. The internal reasons that emerge through reflection allow us to see and act differently because we view such action as consistent with our sense of ourselves, our commitments, projects, and desires. When confronted with an immediate ethical quandary upon which we have not yet reflected and for which we may not be deeply motivated, we may nonetheless have external reasons for acting to promote the well-being of animals – for example, that to do so would respect their independent value or that it would, all things considered, lead to greater good.

There have been disputes within the literature between proponents of these various frameworks that are philosophically interesting, to be sure. It is not clear to me that resolution of these disputes will ultimately help us in addressing the diverse, complex, and pressing ethical issues that we face in our dealings with other animals, however. Rather than attempting

---

[62] Hursthouse 2000: 165–6.

to resolve the disputes in the pages ahead, or promoting one particular normative framework over others, I will instead draw on the resources of these frameworks in discussing the ethical claims animals make on us in a variety of contexts. If we can begin to see other animals as making claims upon us, can make those claims intelligible to ourselves and to others, and can respond in the right ways to those claims, we will become better ethical agents and more robust selves, with a more compassionate – and, I would say, accurate – sense of our place in the animal kingdom.

2 The natural and the normative

Crocodiles are animals who inhabit human nightmares and with good reason. Crocodiles hide below the surface and wait until just the right moment to spring out, toothy mouths ajar, to attack. They are ideal metaphors for the subconscious. They are also truly frightening predators. The late ecofeminist philosopher Val Plumwood had a near fatal encounter with a crocodile and described her terror after enduring a crocodile "death roll." Her description of the attack is horrifying:

> As I pulled the canoe out into the main current, the rain and wind started up again. I had not gone more than five or ten minutes down the channel when, rounding a bend, I saw in midstream what looked like a floating stick – one I did not recall passing on my way up. As the current moved me toward it, the stick developed eyes. A crocodile!... Although I was paddling to miss the crocodile, our paths were strangely convergent. I knew it would be close, but I was totally unprepared for the great blow when it struck the canoe. Again it struck, again and again, now from behind, shuddering the flimsy craft. As I paddled furiously, the blows continued. The unheard of was happening; the canoe was under attack! For the first time, it came to me fully that I was prey. I realized I had to get out of the canoe or risk being capsized.
>
> The bank now presented a high, steep face of slippery mud. The only obvious avenue of escape was a paperbark tree near the muddy bank wall. I made the split-second decision to leap into its lower branches and climb to safety. I steered to the tree and stood up to jump. At the same instant, the crocodile rushed up alongside the canoe, and its beautiful, flecked golden eyes looked straight into mine.... The golden eyes glinted with interest. I tensed for the jump and leapt. Before my foot even tripped the first branch, I had a blurred, incredulous vision of great toothed jaws bursting from the water. Then I was seized between the legs in a red-hot pincer grip and whirled into the suffocating wet darkness.

Few of those who have experienced the crocodile's death roll have lived to describe it. It is, essentially, an experience beyond words of total terror. The crocodile's breathing and heart metabolism are not suited to prolonged struggle, so the roll is an intense burst of power designed to overcome the victim's resistance quickly. The crocodile then holds the feebly struggling prey underwater until it drowns. The roll was a centrifuge of boiling blackness that lasted for an eternity, beyond endurance, but when I seemed all but finished, the rolling suddenly stopped. My feet touched bottom, my head broke the surface, and, coughing, I sucked at air, amazed to be alive. The crocodile still had me in its pincer grip between the legs. I had just begun to weep for the prospects of my mangled body when the crocodile pitched me suddenly into a second death roll.

When the whirling terror stopped again I surfaced again, still in the crocodile's grip next to a stout branch of a large sandpaper fig growing in the water. I grabbed the branch, vowing to let the crocodile tear me apart rather than throw me again into that spinning, suffocating hell. For the first time I realized that the crocodile was growling, as if angry. I braced myself for another roll, but then its jaws simply relaxed; I was free.[1]

In scenes from National Geographic's *Most Amazing Close Encounters* and from the full-length program *Last Feast of the Crocodiles*, crocodiles are shown attacking other animals, in these cases not humans. Most of the attacks result in the animal preyed upon being killed and eaten, although occasionally an animal manages to escape to live temporarily with what are ultimately fatal injuries.

Watching these scenes is like watching a horror movie, only the scenes depicted are real. There was one particular segment that is worth recounting. In this scene, a herd of impala comes to a river to drink.[2] The young impala have not yet learned that danger lurks below the surface of the water. An impetuous young male impala attempts to cross the water and is suddenly attacked by a crocodile who begins to drag the impala, thrashing, under the surface of the muddy river. What happens next is quite surprising. A nearby hippopotamus, noticing the commotion, charges at the crocodile with fierce speed and frees the impala from the grip of death. The hippo nudges the impala out of the water in what looks to be an attempt to save the youngster. The impala stumbles onto land but then collapses. The hippo tries repeatedly to resuscitate the impala, nudging him and trying to prop him up. At one

[1] Plumwood 2000.   [2] www.youtube.com/watch?v=E51DyWl_q0c.

point, the hippo puts the impala's head into her mouth in what looks to be an effort to revive him. Hippopotamuses are herbivores, so the impala would not have been a meal for the hippo. On this particular occasion, the hippo's efforts to resuscitate the impala fail as the impala's injuries from the crocodile attack are too severe. After the impala dies, the hippo wanders away. Almost instantly the crocodile climbs onto the bank to retrieve the carcass and drags the dead impala back to the water to eat it.

There is no way of knowing why the hippo did what she did or how often hippopotamuses exhibit this type of seemingly caring or altruistic behavior in the wild. We do know that, just as crocodiles are predictable predators, hippopotamuses are capable of building cross-species relationships.[3]

These stories, while remarkable in their own right, also raise interesting questions for us to try to answer. Did the crocodile choose to attack Val Plumwood? Did the croc let Plumwood go on purpose? Did the hippo purposely try to help the impala because she recognized the impala was in mortal danger, like the dolphins protecting the swimmers discussed in the last chapter, or was it an instinctual response? If it was instinctual, why did it happen on this occasion, but not on others? Does it make sense to say that what the hippopotamus did in trying to save the impala was good, virtuous, or right? Was what the crocodile did to Plumwood or to the impala wrong? These are questions about the natural and the normative, the topics of this chapter.

The concept of the "natural" is a fraught one; it can mean many different things in different contexts. Too often we think we understand what a claim about what is natural means, but just a little bit of pushing reveals that we may not be particularly clear. Normativity, as we briefly discussed in Chapter 1, also has multiple connotations. It sometimes means what is typical, normal, or expected; it sometimes means what is good; and it sometimes refers to a combination of what is expected and what is good in the form of a prescription for action.

In this chapter we'll explore what is meant by "natural" and what is meant by "normative" in the context of evaluating the grounds of our ethical obligations to other animals. We will begin with a very common skeptical response to the central idea of this book – that we are in ethical relation with other animals and that our attitudes, decisions, and actions have ethical consequences for all of us, humans as well as non-humans. When initially presented with

[3] Hatkoff, et al. 2007.

the idea that other animals matter from a moral point of view, skeptics think, and some even say, "Animals kill, torment, and use other animals, and since they do it, and since we too are animals, why shouldn't we?" Since it is natural for a crocodile to kill and eat an impala, it makes sense to think it is natural for humans to kill and eat crocodiles or, more generally, to do what serves us best, even if that means disregarding the interests and needs of other animals.

Doing what comes naturally

In assessing the skeptic's claim, we first need to determine what it means to act naturally or to do what is natural.

One way we might think of what is natural is in distinction to what is cultural. Natural actions are those that aren't informed or influenced by cultural practices or traditions. This way of understanding the term is popular among certain environmentalists, who tend to see culture as unique to humans and think that our cultures remove us from the natural world. This removal or alienation is thought to be one of the roots of our environmental crises. In order to remedy the problems caused by our separateness from nature, these environmentalists suggest it is important for humans to "get in touch with nature" by eschewing culture. According to this understanding, what is most natural is what is most distant from human culture, civilization, and their influences. The natural is wild, untamed, undomesticated, and free of human concepts and perceptions, including ethical ones.

There are a variety of problems with this dualistic notion of the natural as opposed to the cultural. The first problem is that it seems to be incoherent. If what it means to be natural is being free from human influence, then it appears that humans are "unnatural" by definition. How then are we to make sense of the skeptic's claim that humans are supposed to be "acting naturally" the way other animals do if being human is already acting in unnatural or non-natural ways? Recall those chimpanzees and other tool-using animals we discussed in Chapter 1. Primatologists and ethologists suggest that some of their behaviors are "cultural." There are different sorts of traditions and practices that vary between populations that aren't strictly explicable in terms of ecological variations in their habitat ranges. According to these observations, cultural innovation and the transmission of cultural practices seem perfectly natural. So nature and culture aren't contrary to one another, and humans and other animals may engage in both "natural" and "cultural" behaviors.

The idea that nature is distinct from culture can also be seen as self-defeating. If there were an imperative to "get back to nature," it would result from human conceptual and ethical reflection, which, according to the dualistic conception under consideration, is unnatural. This conception of nature, as William Cronin has so forcefully argued in "Getting Back to the Wrong Nature: Why We Need to End our Love Affair with Wilderness," rests on a profound misunderstanding. Cronin writes, "Viewing nature and ourselves in such stark, absolute terms leaves us little hope of discovering what an ethical, sustainable, honorable human place in nature might actually look like."[4] There is no way to value what is natural, because according to this understanding of what it means to be natural, the very process of valuing ends up devaluing nature.

So understanding nature as distinct from culture isn't particularly sensible. Another proposal for understanding what it means to be doing what is "natural" is to think of natural behavior as synonymous with instinctual behavior. The idea here is that when the crocodile attacks the impala the croc is acting on instinct, and the skeptic's claim, if we understand natural to mean instinctual, is that it is instinctual for us to use other animals to serve our ends. But what exactly is instinct? The notion of "instinct" has been subject to almost as much conceptual challenge as has "nature," and it may be that replacing "natural" with "instinctual" will not be particularly illuminating. Historically, there were debates among psychologists and ethologists about what instincts were. Some saw instincts as automatic reactions to specific stimuli; others saw them as adaptable motivations that underlie behavior; and still others saw instincts as heritable systems "of co-ordination within the nervous system as a whole, which when activated find expression in behaviour culminating in a fixed action pattern."[5] Sometimes the term "instinctual" has been used interchangeably with the term "innate." Yet, here again, we may be exchanging one slippery term for another as there is a tremendous debate about what constitutes "innateness."

Commenting on innateness, ethologist Patrick Bateson identifies at least six meanings for the term: "present at birth; a behavioral difference caused by a genetic difference; adapted over the course of evolution; unchanging throughout development; shared by all members of a species; and not

---

[4] Cronin 1996a: 3.   [5] Thorpe 1950 as cited in Griffiths 2004: 614.

learned."[6] Each of these different meanings has very different implications, and, as Paul Griffiths has argued, "the concept of innateness conflates a number of independent biological properties and is thus a confusing and unhelpful notion with which to understand behavioral or cognitive development."[7] So when it comes to trying to understand what counts as natural behavior, relying on some construal of innateness or instinct has not proven explanatorily useful. We are merely replacing one vague concept, the natural, with reductive and equally vague concepts.

In the last quarter century, developments in the field of evolutionary developmental biology (what is called "evo-devo") suggest we adopt a more-integrative, less-reductive understanding of the nature of development where genes and their environments are interacting to affect phenotypic, including behavioral, characteristics of the organism. In other words, an evo-devo approach maintains that there aren't traits or behaviors that can be explained purely by innate or hardwired instincts; science does not support the view that underlies the old "nature–nurture" debates. Developmental systems theorist Susan Oyama puts the point forcefully:

> To call something biological (or genetic, natural, or innate) is clearly not just to make a bare scientific statement. It is also to pronounce on the relevance of experience and the conditions of life . . . The same is true for the contrasting terms: cultural, acquired, environmental. If something is biological, it is reasoned, it is physical, preprogrammed and controlled from the inside; while learning is an accident of personal history, a product of mind, not body. This echo of an ancient dualism should raise suspicions . . . the traditional nature–nurture categories are incoherent. I suggest . . . we free ourselves from the whole set of interlaced conceptual habits that keeps these disputes going.[8]

All this debate about the meaning of the terms natural, instinctual, or innate doesn't erase the possibility that there is something meaningful that the skeptic is trying to say. There are some behaviors that seem to be typical to a species. As we briefly discussed in the last chapter and will return to in Chapter 5, accurately interpreting the behavior of other animals is an important part of understanding what their interests are and how our actions may impact their abilities to satisfy those interests. Recognizing species-typical behaviors, then, is an important part of understanding other animals. So, to return to

---

[6] Bateson 1991: 21–2 as cited in Griffiths, et al. 2009: 605.
[7] Griffiths 2002: 70–85.   [8] Oyama 2007.

our skeptic's claim, perhaps what he means when he says that it is natural for humans to use other animals to serve our ends is that it is part of our species-typical behavioral repertoire, much as it is for the crocodile. Using other species for food, clothing, protection, or even entertainment is something that we, as a species, evolved to do. As a couple of skeptics put it, "it is an evolutionary necessity to regard one's own kind as more important than other species."[9] That we evolved to want to further our own species' interests, at the expense of members of other species, if need be, may very well be what the skeptic means when he says it is natural for us to use other animals.

There are two issues raised by this particular version of the skeptic's challenge. First is the issue of understanding what it means to say that a species evolved to perform certain behaviors or to have certain attitudes. Second, even if there were a way to establish that performing certain behaviors or having certain attitudes was natural or a product of evolutionary forces, we need to ask whether having a preference for one's own species, what has been called "speciesism," is justified. In other words, does the natural justify the normative?

Species and speciesism

You probably won't be surprised, at this point in the discussion, to learn that there are multiple and contested meanings of the concept of "species" and that whether a particular population of organisms is classified as a species may change, even quickly, so particular individuals who are currently members of one species may later become members of a new species.[10] Conversely, individuals who were once members of different species may be classified as a single species. Our understanding of species relies on various sorts of judgments based on the reasons we need the classification and how such a classification will help to organize particular inquiries and practices. Species categorizations are not, strictly speaking, fixed by nature but rather are constructed by

---

[9] Nicholl & Russell 2001: 165.

[10] Karen Strier wrote: "I have been studying the same group of monkeys, known as northern muriquis, in a small forest in southeastern Brazil for nearly 28 years. When I began my research they were called *Brachyteles arachnoides*. Subsequently, and within the lifetimes of many of the individuals in my original study group, they were reclassified as a new species, *B. hypoxanthus*, to distinguish them (as northern muriquis) from the southern muriqui, which has retained the original Latin name." Strier 2010.

us to understand the natural world. Without going further into the fascinating debate about the species concept here, let us posit that "species," as well as "species-typical behaviors," are not simply biologically or naturally given and are not necessarily immutable, although they are based, in part, on evolved biological properties, some of which may be intrinsic and others relational. Given that species is not a biologically determinate classification, species are not, in evolutionary terms, what natural selection operates on – rather it is populations or groups, if that.[11] If species is a relatively arbitrary unit in evolutionary terms, it does not make sense to suggest, as the skeptic has, that a preference for members of one's own species is a product of evolution.

In addition, both empirical and historical examinations show that it simply is not the case that members of the same lineage, species, or population do prefer or protect their own. Ethological studies have established that members of the same species, conspecifics, often compete fiercely with one another to survive, and in some cases will kill their own kind. Some animals even kill their own siblings. Great egret chicks are known to peck their youngest sibling to death and then push him out of the nest.[12] Many mammals, from rats to primates, practice infanticide on conspecifics. Most individuals appear to be concerned with their own survival, and possibly the survival of their offspring or other members of their immediate group, not the survival of their species as a whole. This is also the case among humans. The history of our own kind is full of examples of mass murders, wars, and genocides. Humans, like other social animals, are particularly adept at identifying in-groups and out-groups and granting respect and protection to those in their own group, and exhibiting contempt and disregard for others, no matter if they are members of our species or others.

But nature isn't always red in tooth and claw. There are less frequent, but regularly documented cases in which members of one species help or protect

[11] There are debates about units of selection (e.g., whether genes, cells, organisms, and/or populations ultimately evolve) among biologists and philosophers. For a philosophically rich discussion, see Godfrey-Smith 2009. There are some, most notably David Sloan Wilson and Eliott Sober, who argue that selection can be understood to operate on groups, and the late Steven Jay Gould, who argued for species selection. See, for a start, Wilson 1993 and Lieberman & Vrba 2005.

[12] My colleague Barry Chernoff told me about the case of siblicide among armadillos who are actually genetically identical twins. So when one armadillo kills her sibling she is, in a sense, killing herself. He also mentioned that male fish, who look after the young, on occasion will be forced to kill the mother as she is threatening to kill and eat her young.

members of another species – as was the case with the dolphins discussed at the beginning of the last chapter and the hippopotamus discussed earlier. The struggle for survival may pit one animal against another, but it also involves animals cooperating against obstacles and hardships in their environments. Sometimes this will bring members of different species together for mutual advantage.

The capacity to identify and favor those within one's own group, and to deny resources to or attack those who are outsiders, undoubtedly conferred some evolutionary advantage on those who exercised this capacity. Yet the fact that a capacity is evolutionarily advantageous does not have a direct bearing on whether or not we humans (or other animals), here and now, are ethically justified in continuing to invoke that capacity. At certain points in our history, some humans may have experienced greater reproductive success relative to other humans because the males raped and impregnated the females. That this practice generated an evolutionary advantage to the group that practiced rape doesn't justify rape. The moral permissibility of exercising a particular capacity, or engaging in a particular action, is not determined by the evolutionary history or the success of the use of the capacity. As the late Stephen Jay Gould wrote, "nature favors none and offers no guidelines. The facts of nature cannot provide moral guidance in any case."[13]

One of the capacities that humans have, and perhaps other animals, as well, is the ability to make decisions about what behavior to engage in and what course of action to follow. We may make bad choices – eat or drink too much, have unsafe sex, smoke cigarettes, destroy our environments – but we are not always destined to act on our bad choice. We can change our behavior. Appeals to nature do not ethically justify various actions, including the use of other animals, as we'll see. Much of what is thought to be natural behavior is, in fact, conventional behavior, behavior that we can, and should, hold up to normative scrutiny and ask whether there are reasons to refrain from doing certain things that we thought, before reflection, were permissible.

There are many human behaviors that feel utterly natural, but, as we have just seen, it is sometimes difficult to explicate what lies behind that feeling. Throughout human history, in-groups have often justified discriminatory and violent behaviors toward out-groups by appeals to what is natural. The history of genocides, too horrible to recount here, contain multiple examples of

---

[13] Gould 1997: 13.

attitudes and rhetoric in which those being destroyed are likened to animals, a comparison that justifies their destruction.

In the 1970s, Richard Ryder suggested that the species boundary was being used to identify who is "in" and who is "out," and he coined the term "speciesism" to denote this type of prejudice. Shortly thereafter, Peter Singer popularized the term as being comparable to racism and sexism. He argued that movements to end oppression often begin by uncovering a basic idea and set of practices that seem natural and inevitable that, when subjected to careful scrutiny, turn out to be unjustifiably discriminatory.

> Racists violate the principle of equality by giving greater weight to the interests of members of their own race when there is a clash between their interests and the interests of those of another race ... Similarly, speciesists allow the interests of their own species to override the greater interests of members of other species. The pattern is identical in each case.[14]

When we consider the reasons that people have given for denying equality to non-whites, to women, and to gay men, lesbians, and transgendered people, we often see that the prejudice is naturalized. One need only recall the debates over gay marriage to illuminate how this is so. Much of the popular and legal rhetoric employed by opponents of recognizing gay marriage was infused with claims about the "unnaturalness" of gay and lesbian relationships and arguments that socially endorsing such behavior by allowing gay people to marry would legitimize this unnatural behavior. Attempts to disguise animus against non-heterosexual people by naturalizing heterosexuality, though often politically successful, do not withstand the demands for equal respect. Similarly, Ryder and Singer argue that invoking species membership in order to deny the moral claims of those who are not members of the "in" species amounts to unjustified prejudice.

Discrimination on the basis of skin color, gender, sexual orientation, or being able-bodied is thought to be prejudicial, because these are not characteristics that matter when it comes to making moral claims or demanding moral attention. That one is a woman or in a wheelchair should not bear on whether an individual's interests matter from an ethical point of view. Species membership, it has been argued, is also morally irrelevant when it comes to determining who can make moral claims. If an individual's life can

[14] Singer 1990: 9

go better or worse for her, by her own lights; if she has interests and desires, the satisfaction of which will contribute to her well-being; and my behavior can impact her life for better or worse, then my failing to consider how my actions affect that individual would be morally irresponsible. If a child runs out into the street, and I purposely fail to stop my car because the child was Asian or a boy or wore leg-braces, I would rightly be judged a monster. Similarly, if I fail to stop my car and purposely run over a cat, I will not be excused by saying, "it was only a cat." These are individuals who have interests in not being run over by cars, and when I fail to consider these interests I put my very capacity to act morally in question. My interests in getting to my destination faster, or not being bothered to stop, do not obviously outweigh the interests of those who inadvertently cross my path.

Sexism and racism involve actions and attitudes (either conscious or not) that elevate the interests of one's own gender or race over the interests of another gender or race, merely because the sexist favors his gender and the racist favors his race, over others. Similarly, speciesism involves actions and attitudes that elevate human interests above the interests of any other species, because humans favor humans over others and think of humans as superior. Speciesist actions and attitudes are prejudicial, because there is no prima facie reason for preferring the interests of beings like me, or of those belonging to my group, to the interests of those who are different. I happen to have been born a human female in the US, but I could have been born a male in Australia or a chimpanzee in Africa. It is just a bit of luck that I was born me, and it is no more interesting from a moral point of view, than the fact that I have five fingers on each hand, including opposable thumbs. I'm happy I have the hands I do. But, having hands like mine doesn't give me more of a claim to moral attention than those who don't have hands like mine, and it doesn't justify my devaluing the interests of those who have different sorts of hands. Species membership is a morally irrelevant characteristic, and, given our discussion above, classification of the species to which I belong seems even less important, given that it is a matter of convention, rather than something irrevocably or naturally fixed.

Of course, that I am a human and not a chimpanzee has implications for how I am treated. If I were a chimpanzee, my particular interests would be different. I would undoubtedly want to live a quite different, more active sort of life. Ideally, I would want to be in a tropical forest with lots of fresh fruits and vegetation and other chimpanzees. A chimpanzee's interests in living a good life for her are no less morally important than my human interests simply because they are not human interests. Difference does not justify disregard.

Attending to the specific interests of other individuals whose interests matter from a moral point of view will require attending to both the biological and the social facts about those individuals. Although some of the morally relevant facts might be gleaned from species membership, many of them won't be so apparent. That an individual is a human may not tell us everything we need to know about how to treat that individual, and the same will be true of members of other species. For example, we hold some humans accountable for their actions in a way that we forgive others for the same actions. A paradigm example is children – when a toddler hurts the dog or another child, we don't think the toddler has done something morally wrong. Even if the toddler were to cause the death of another, say by picking up a loaded gun and shooting his sister, we would certainly find that tragic, but we wouldn't say that the child was a monster in the way that we might the adult who purposely runs over a cat. This is because a toddler has not yet developed the skills necessary to understand right from wrong and to make a decision about how to act based on that understanding. A human child, much like the crocodile, is acting without reflecting. Both lack the capacity to reflect on their actions and, thus, cannot decide to act differently. Because they cannot decide to do otherwise, we do not hold them ethically responsible for their actions. In philosophical parlance, the human child and the crocodile are not persons.

Humans and persons

Philosophers make a distinction between humans and persons. This may seem somewhat odd and contrary to common usage as we ordinarily think of the two as synonymous. It is understandable to be reluctant to accept this as a meaningful distinction on first gloss. As one scholar has pointed out, "Philosophers have made rather heavy weather of the concept of a person. Heavy weather can make interesting philosophy but it does not necessarily lead to true, clear or even any answers. If philosophically interesting conceptions of personhood lead to false and obnoxious conclusions then in the end we will have to give up those conceptions."[15] Indeed, there are a number of

[15] Teichman 1985: 176.

philosophical distinctions that don't make a difference, or at least much of a difference, and some philosophical distinctions may very well be offensive but they may nonetheless be important. The case of defining persons separate from humans is central in the context of discussions about our relationships with non-human animals and arguments for making the distinction play an important historical and conceptual role in discussions of moral status and moral obligations. After analyzing these arguments, I hope you will see that this particular distinction is a meaningful one. Yet, the reluctance to accept it, particularly a reluctance based on a worry that the distinction is "offensive," is also worth considering, and we will discuss this later in the chapter.

A human is a member of the species *Homo sapiens*. Since there is not one singular definition of species, let's use a reproductive isolation definition for species for the purposes of discussion. This will help us to see humans as distinct from aardvarks and apple trees, chimpanzees and cycads. Humans come in different types and sizes and have a wide range of abilities, but we have the same ontogeny; we share a distinctive developmental history. *Homo sapiens* is the product of the fusion of two human gametes that then develops in a uterine environment.[16] Most other mammals are the product of the fusion of gametes from two members of their species and spend some amount of time in a uterus, although it needn't necessarily be the uterus of the same species.[17] Some mammals, such as the platypus, lay eggs. Other mammals, such as wombats and wallabies, are born in almost embryonic form and develop in their mother's pouch. These reproductive links – that humans are born of humans and not other types of organisms – allow us to distinguish humans from other species. Giraffes are born of and give birth to other giraffes. Hens lay eggs that hatch chickens, not cheetahs. Dandelion seeds produce dandelions, not daisies.

The fact that each member of a species is reproductively linked to other members of the species, as we've discussed, is not in itself interesting from

---

[16] Until fairly recently it made sense to say that humans develop in a woman's body, but given the fluidity of gender and the fact that some people who were born with female reproductive organs identify as men and some of those men have given birth to children, it is more accurate to say that humans, at least until technology becomes more advanced, develop in uterine environments, whether those belong to individuals identifying as "women," "men," or some other gender category.

[17] For example, as the result of developments in reproductive technologies, including cloning, surrogate mothers can be a different species from the developing infant.

an ethical point of view. Just as other kinds of reproductive information, such as the fact that dandelions reproduce asexually or that gibbons are monogamous, don't tell us anything about how we should treat these organisms, whether they have obligations or duties, or what obligations and duties we might have toward them in light of such information. Reproductive practices, expectations, and contexts may raise ethical issues; in humans there are a variety of ethical issues that arise in the context of assisted reproduction, for example, and in other animals there is a significant ethical issue that arises in the context of captive breeding that we will discuss in Chapter 5. But the biological facts of reproduction, that humans reproduce with other humans and that seahorses reproduce with other seahorses, for example, don't pose ethical issues in themselves.

That one is "human" identifies a descriptive feature of that being; that one is a "person" identifies a normative feature. The notion of "personhood" is used to identify the value or worth of someone, and it has also been used to identify who has "rights" and who is the subject of ethical duties and obligations. Not all humans have rights or duties, and some other than human beings may have worth. Distinguishing humans from persons marks these ethical differences.

This distinction between humans and persons appears in a number of philosophical discussions both historical and contemporary. Immanuel Kant posited two important capacities, rationality and self-awareness, that were associated with persons and distinguished persons from "things." He wrote:

> every rational being exists as an end in himself and not merely as a means to be arbitrarily used by this or that will . . . Beings whose existence depends not on our will but on nature have, nevertheless, if they are not rational beings, only a relative value as means and are therefore called things. On the other hand, rational beings are called persons inasmuch as their nature already marks them out as ends in themselves.[18]

In his *Lectures on Anthropology* Kant wrote, "The fact that the human being can have the representation 'I' raises him infinitely above all the other beings on earth. By this he is a person . . . that is, a being altogether different in rank and dignity from things, such as irrational animals, with which one may deal and dispose at one's discretion."[19] Similarly, John Locke defined a person as

---

[18] As cited in Wood 1998.   [19] Kant 1798: 7, 127.

a "thinking intelligent being that has reason and reflection and can consider itself as itself, the same thinking thing, in different times and places."[20] In more contemporary language, we might say that a Lockean person is someone who has certain psychological capacities – cognition, self-awareness, and episodic memory. While Locke's view of personhood is primarily aimed at identifying what capacities are needed in order to classify an individual as a person, Kant's view of personhood has stronger normative implications. Only persons seem to matter morally on Kant's view.

For Kant, it appears that non-rational beings who do not have a self-conception – non-persons – are mere things. But some humans lack rationality and do not have a self-conception. Fetuses, newborns, and probably even toddlers don't yet have the concept of themselves as themselves, distinct from others, and thus wouldn't be considered persons, even though they are humans. The same is true of a human in a permanent vegetative state. The distinction between humans and persons has become a central one in the bioethics literature. Whether we have duties to humans before they are persons (at the beginning of life) and what sorts of obligations we have to humans when they are no longer persons (after significant brain injuries or at the end of life) are some of the most pressing questions for health care providers and policymakers. Kant's view would not allow us to recognize that there are important ethical questions to address here. Similarly, Kant's view would have us deny most, but maybe not all, other animals moral concern. This seems highly counterintuitive.[21]

---

[20] Locke 1690: Bk. II, Ch. 27, sect. 9.

[21] There have been arguments about how to get around this counterintuitive problem for Kant. There are three possible responses. One is to suggest that non-persons are morally considerable indirectly. Though Kant believed that animals were mere things, it appears he did not genuinely believe we could dispose of them any way we wanted. In the *Lectures on Ethics* he makes it clear that we have indirect duties to animals, duties that are not toward them, but in regard to them, insofar as our treatment of them can affect our duties to persons. And one could argue the same would be true of those human beings who are not persons. We disrespect our humanity when we act in inhumane ways toward non-persons, whatever their species. But this too is unsatisfying – it fails to capture the independent wrong that is being done to the non-person. When someone rapes a woman in a coma, or whips a severely brain-damaged child, or sets a cat on fire, they are not simply disrespecting humanity or themselves as representatives of it, it can be argued that they are wronging these non-persons. So, a second way to avoid the counterintuitive conclusion is to argue that such non-persons stand in the proper relations to "rational nature" such that they should be thought of as morally considerable. Allen Wood (1998)

While we may be tempted to reject the very notion of the distinction between humans and persons because of this counterintuitive result, we can also accept a general, more descriptive understanding of what it means to be a person, more like Locke's view, without accepting the normative implications of Kant's view.

Some humans may not be persons and some non-humans may well be persons, but the distinction itself doesn't say anything about what this means from an ethical point of view if we don't accept Kant's perspective. Before we turn to the question of what ethical status persons and non-persons have, let's first briefly examine which other animals might be persons. As we discussed in the last chapter, the cognitive capacities of many other animals are well documented. There is also growing evidence that many non-humans have self-awareness and episodic memory. One of the ways that psychologists try to establish whether or not an individual has self-awareness is by testing to see whether that individual can recognize him- or herself in a mirror. Great apes are able to recognize themselves, whereas most of the monkeys tested are not. Studies with dolphins, elephants, pigs, and pigeons have suggested that they can pass the mirror test, but dogs, cats, and young human children don't recognize themselves in mirrors.[22] Episodic memory is more difficult to test, but in one of the more remarkable studies, episodic-like memory has been found in scrub jays by Nicky Clayton and her colleagues. Episodic memory involves recalling "where" a unique event or episode took place, "what" occurred during the episode, and "when" the episode happened. In her experimental work, Clayton found that these food-storing jays remember "what," "when," and "where" food items are cached in experiments in which the birds are allowed to recover perishable "wax worms" and non-perishable peanuts, "which they had previously cached in visuospatially distinct sites. Jays searched preferentially for fresh wax worms, their favoured food, when allowed to recover them shortly after caching. However, they rapidly learned

argues in this way and suggests that all beings that potentially have a rational nature, or who virtually have it, or who have had it, or who have part of it, or who have the necessary conditions of it, what he calls "the infrastructure of rational nature," should be directly morally considerable. Insofar as a being stands in this relation to rational nature, they are the kinds of beings that can be wronged. The third way has been proposed by Christine Korsgaard (2004), who argues that though only persons can make moral demands on other persons, what we demand is that our animal natures be respected. I discuss Korsgaard's view in the next section.

[22] See Broom, et al. 2009 for pigs and Reiss & Marino 2001 for dolphins.

to avoid searching for worms after a longer interval during which the worms had decayed."[23] Clayton's observations suggest that the birds "form integrated memories about what happened where and when, rather than encoding the information separately. Furthermore, the jays can also remember whether another individual was present at the time of caching, and if so, who was watching when."[24] If jays have a self-conception, then they might count as persons.

So there are human persons and non-human persons, human non-persons and non-human non-persons. Of course, more empirical work and further conceptual refinement of the definition of personhood will help us to figure out what sorts of beings, with what sorts of capacities, fall into what category, and thus, what specific moral claims and responsibilities they will, in fact, have. Even before we have definitive answers about "where to draw the lines," as it were, we can still explore what general ethical obligations or attitudes we should have to those who are not persons but who still deserve our moral attention.

Moral agents and moral patients

Some philosophers have marked the normative distinction between persons and non-persons by indicating that persons are "moral agents" and non-persons are "moral patients." Moral agents as persons have certain capacities that allow them to make reflective choices about their actions and to attend to those who may not be able to make such choices but who nonetheless have lives that will be affected, for better or worse, by our actions. These latter non-persons are moral patients; they are the recipients of moral attention and concern, but they do not have the moral responsibilities that moral agents, as persons, do. Because moral patients lack certain capacities, there may be certain things that it is not wrong to do to them, that would be wrong if these very same actions were done to persons. One of the capacities that persons or moral agents are generally thought to have, following Locke, is a sense of themselves as existing over time. Non-persons or moral patients lack this capacity. So, painlessly killing a non-person who has no conscious interest or desire to continue living is not, all things considered,

---

[23] Clayton & Dickinson 1998: 272–4. See also Clayton, et al. 2003.
[24] Clayton, et al. 2007: R190.

wrong in the way that killing a person who does have an explicit desire to continue to exist would be, other things being equal. Similarly, persons are autonomous, and, thus, denying them their freedom would be ethically problematic. In the case of many non-persons who lack autonomy, denying them freedom may actually be the right thing to do from an ethical perspective. We will talk about the issues of killing and liberty in greater depth in the chapters ahead.

For now, it is important to see that the scope of ethical attention extends over a broad range of beings, all of whom have valuable capacities and interests as we discussed in the last chapter: they are alive and have bodies that experience pleasures and pains and can suffer from violence, neglect, or abuse; they have emotions, desires, likes, and dislikes; and they are engaged in the world in a variety of ways, some which are enriching and some which are debilitating. If you are a being whose life can go better or worse, then you are a proper object of moral attention. A subset of attention-worthy beings has additional capabilities and interests as well as obligations and responsibilities. Moral agents not only have interests in living lives that are good for them by their own lights, full of enriching experiences, pleasurable activities, and satisfying projects, but they also have ethical obligations that arise, in part, because they have the capacity to reason about their actions and alter their behaviors accordingly. Moral agents can form intentions about their actions; are causally responsible for actions and can be blamed or praised for them; are able to make judgments about rightness and wrongness, both of their own conduct and of the conduct of other agents; and can construct and follow norms or moral principles.

The moral universe, as it were, thus can be said to have two levels: a level that contains moral agents, actors who are responsible for doing the right thing; and a level that contains moral patients, those to whom right or wrong actions are directed, but who may or may not be moral agents themselves. Someone who lacks the capacities of personhood will always be at the level of a moral patient. But the levels are not exclusive. In certain contexts, persons can be moral patients too – for example, when they are the ones acted upon by moral agents, when they are benefited or harmed by others, or when they temporarily lose their capacities for reason and reflection. Similarly, upon changes in the abilities of a moral patient, our understanding of those abilities, or changes in the context in which moral agency is expressed, moral patients may turn out to be moral agents some of the time.

This two-level view of morality can be identified in both utilitarian thinking and in the thinking of some contemporary Kantians.

For example, Peter Singer's "preference utilitarianism" allows for differential ethical responses to agents and patients, persons and non-persons. Singer believes that we must take into account the consequences of our actions on all those who experience pleasure or pain as a result of that action, and that accounting requires that like interests be treated equally, no matter who has them. Sentient beings have interests, particularly interests in experiencing pleasure and avoiding pain. Since most humans and non-human animals are sentient beings who are capable of feeling pleasure and pain, the happiness and suffering of most humans and other animals should be taken into account. Things – like rocks, plants, and eco-systems – are not taken into account. So the boundary of moral concern is drawn around the group of beings who are sentient. However, Singer is concerned not simply with interests in avoiding pain and experiencing pleasure, but also with interests and desires that are projected into the future. So, within the sphere of moral concern, there are two classes of beings: those who project their desires into the future and those who do not have that capacity. When you or I have our future desires frustrated, the disappointment and mental suffering that may result is different than it would be for a being who doesn't have a concept of the future. Without a concept of time, or of existence into the future, one cannot suffer a particular kind of harm, that of having one's future preferences thwarted. Singer's preference utilitarianism thus judges actions not solely by their tendency to maximize happiness and minimize pain, but also by their role in promoting interests or satisfying preferences (and avoiding violations of interests or frustration of preferences).

Christine Korsgaard, who works in the Kantian tradition, has argued that what we are calling moral agents face "the problem of normativity" because of the reflective structure of our consciousness.[25] We can, and often do, think about our desires and ask ourselves, "Are these desires reasons for action? Do these impulses represent the kind of things I want to act according to?" Our reflective capacities allow us, *and* require us, to step back from our mere impulses in order to determine when and whether to act on them. In stepping back, we gain a certain distance from which we can answer these questions and solve the problem of normativity. We decide whether to treat our desires

---

[25] She uses the term "human" when she is describing what we are calling "persons."

as reasons for action based on our conceptions of ourselves, on our "practical identities." When we determine whether we should take a particular desire as a reason to act, we are engaging in a further level of reflection, a level that requires an endorsable description of ourselves. This endorsable description of ourselves, this practical identity, is a necessary moral identity because, without it, we cannot view our lives as worth living or our actions as worth doing. According to Korsgaard, moral agents have a conception of what it is we ought to do and what other agents ought to do. Persons are aware of the grounds of our beliefs and actions as grounds; non-persons or moral patients lack this awareness.

Korsgaard sees the difference between those with normative, rational capacities and those without as a big difference. But, unlike Kant, who thought that only the former can have obligations **and** make moral claims, she argues that those without normative, rational capacities share certain "natural" capacities with persons, and these natural capacities are often the content of the moral demands that persons make on each other. She writes:

> *what* we demand, when we demand . . . recognition, is that our *natural* concerns – the objects of our natural desires and interests and affections – be accorded the status of values, values that must be respected as far as possible by others. And many of those natural concerns – the desire to avoid pain is an obvious example – spring from our animal nature, not from our rational nature.[26]

What moral agents construct as valuable and normatively binding is not only our rational or autonomous capacities, but the needs and desires we have as living, embodied beings. Insofar as these needs and desires are valuable for agents, the ability to experience similar needs and desires in patients should also be valued. As a result, moral agents have duties to moral patients.

The two-level view of the moral universe – one that recognizes the moral claims of agents and patients as springing from the same source, and the duties and responsibilities of agents that emerge as a result of their status as persons – appears in competing ethical theories. These theories will differ when it comes to determining how to adjudicate conflicts of values and what particularly constitutes right action. As we'll see when discussing specific issues, such as experimentation on other animals and conflicts that arise in

[26] Korsgaard 2007: 9.

assessing various strategies for addressing threats to wild animals, there will be a good deal of substantive disagreement among these theories. Nonetheless, it is reassuring to note that there is an emerging common vision that humans and other animals populate the moral universe.

The argument from marginal cases

Despite this apparent common ground about how and why we recognize our moral obligations to other animals, there have been complex, often passionate, debates about the characterization I have been making about the sphere of moral concern. In particular, there has been reluctance from some quarters to accept the distinction between humans and persons. Those who support the distinction often use it to make the case for greater ethical regard and better treatment for other animals, and they sometimes invoke what has been called the "Argument from Marginal Cases," or the AMC, for short. The AMC goes something like this:

1. Some humans lack certain capacities or characteristics that are typical of normal human adults (e.g., intentionality, self-awareness, memory, imagination, a sense of existing over time). They are non-persons.
2. Many other animals also lack these capacities or characteristics (although, as we have seen, some other animals may have them). They, too, are non-persons.
3. Our general ethical attitudes about and conduct toward the humans mentioned in 1 are dramatically different from attitudes about and conduct toward the comparable non-human animals mentioned in 2. (For example, it is generally accepted that we use other animals for food or in lethal scientific experiments. It is thought to be monstrous to even consider the use of infants or severely mentally impaired individuals in such ways.)
4. Since there aren't any morally relevant capacities or characteristics that distinguish humans mentioned in 1 from the non-humans mentioned in 2, our general ethical attitudes are inconsistent. (Species membership, as we discussed earlier, even if we had an operational definition of species, is not a morally relevant characteristic.)
5. It is inconsistent to treat individuals mentioned in 1 differently than we treat individuals mentioned in 2. To be consistent, we must either find it

ethically permissible to think about and treat humans mentioned in
1 as we currently do non-humans, or we must think it is ethically
impermissible to think about and treat the non-humans mentioned in 2
as we do.

While proponents of the AMC generally use the argument to ground claims
that we should expand the sphere of those who deserve ethical attention, the
conclusion has led some to worry that the argument will diminish the respect
we have for humans who are not persons. And this worry is not unwarranted.
As Eva Kittay has noted:

> Personhood in the past has also been used less capaciously to exclude specific
> humans: women, slaves, Jews, certain racial groups, the disabled – those who,
> for one reason or another, were believed unworthy or incapable of rationality
> and self-governance. As current disputes over the moral personhood of fetuses
> and very premature neonates attest, personhood has been, and continues to
> be, a contested category.
>
>   What endows these controversies with urgency are the real-life stakes, for
> personhood marks the moral threshold above which equal respect for the
> intrinsic value of an individual's life is required and the requirements of
> justice are operative and below which only relative interest has moral
> weight.[27]

The conclusion of the AMC allows that if we are to be fully consistent in
our ethical reasoning, to avoid acting on prejudice, and to strive to treat like
cases alike, we must change our attitudes and practices. But this can go in two
directions: either to grant ethical considerations to those who fall outside the
human species boundary and who fall outside the boundary of the category
of person, or to deny ethical consideration to anyone other than persons –
that is, to accept something like the counterintuitive conclusion that Kant
seemed to be advancing.

   In order to prevent the possibility of excluding some humans who are on
the margins of personhood from direct ethical consideration, two types of
responses have been mounted. One challenges the notion that moral consideration rests on the possession of certain intrinsic properties, arguing instead
that we ought to take into account the social relations in which individuals
are embedded. The other response is based on the offensiveness of the AMC

---

[27] Kittay 2005: 101.

and the dangers associated with comparing some humans with animals. Let's consider each of these responses in turn.[28]

Social relations

The ability to decide between eating pizza or stir-fried veggies, to enjoy the warmth of the sun on a crisp spring day, to laugh when being tickled, to enjoy a Beethoven piano concerto is based on the possession of intrinsic properties particular to individuals with certain types of perceptual and cognitive capacities. As we have been discussing the occupants of the moral universe in this chapter and the last, we have explored a range of such capacities. One of the reasons that philosophers tend to examine intrinsic capacities in determining who matters from an ethical point of view is that by focusing on the capacities an individual possesses, extrinsic considerations such as popularity, usefulness to others, political expediency, and social prejudice can be set aside. If I am the sort of being whose life can go well if I have the company of good friends and enough chocolate, I should not be denied the opportunity to spend time with friends and eat chocolate just because I am Jewish or a woman. Belonging to a politically marginalized or unpopular group is not a morally relevant social fact about me. No one should be denied the possibility of exercising their capacities and satisfying their interests simply because of inegalitarian social conventions or discriminatory traditions. These sorts of relational properties have a long history of being used to exclude members of "out" groups, and appeals to such relational properties have led to ethically unacceptable practices and policies. It is interesting, then, that recently some philosophers have challenged the AMC, because it is focused on intrinsic properties rather than relational ones. These philosophers argue that some social relations must be taken into account.

Of course, to be able to exercise the deliberative capacities I just mentioned – to have access to pizza or pizza-making ingredients, to be able to listen to Beethoven, and to be with friends – presupposes that the individuals who are in a position to exercise their capacities are embedded in social relations. We wouldn't know what pizza or Beethoven or friendship was without our human

---

[28] It is quite interesting that these arguments are raised in particular against those who argue for extending concern for sentient beings (philosophers like Peter Singer and Jeff McMahan, who are consequentialists) when it seems that the worries would be just as troubling for Kantians.

communities enabling us to understand that there are choices to make and providing us with a range of things to choose over. Indeed, many (some might argue all) of the choices we make to satisfy our interests are influenced and informed by our social relations. My sense of myself as someone whose life can go better or worse for me in particular ways is a product of my social relations. If I had a different upbringing, for example, I might not find satisfaction in what I now find satisfying. Before we persons came to be the kinds of beings who could more or less autonomously exercise our capacities, we were dependent upon a network of care to help us to satisfy our most basic needs. In all of these senses, the individual capacities we have are necessarily embedded in social relations. I think to some extent this is true of all mammals, and particularly social mammals. Our "animal nature," to use Korsgaard's term, is inherently a social nature. Infants cannot survive without caretakers, and developing children require others to help them understand and navigate their worlds.

But this is not the only sense of social relations that critics of the AMC are invoking. For those who object to the AMC, there are species-specific social relations that are thought to make a difference from an ethical perspective. A human person's normative commitments do not emerge solely from their intrinsic psychological capacities; rather they are constructed and made meaningful in social relations with other humans. As Elizabeth Anderson has suggested, "Principles of justice [one example of a normative commitment] cannot be derived simply from a consideration of the intrinsic capacities of moral patients. Their shape also depends on the nature of moral agents, the natural and social relations they do and can have with moral patients, and the social meanings such relations have."[29] To illustrate, she has us consider an individual with a profound case of Alzheimer's, someone who is clearly a moral patient, as this individual is unable to recognize herself or others, to reason, or to care for herself. Anderson argues that this individual's dignity would be violated if she was:

> not properly toileted and decently dressed in clean clothes, her hair combed, her face and nose wiped, and so forth. These demands have only partially to do with matters of health and hygiene. They are, more fundamentally, matters of making the body fit for human society for presentation to others. Human beings need to live with other humans, but cannot do so if those

[29] Anderson 2004: 280.

others cannot relate to them as human. And this specifically human relationship requires that the human body be dignified, protected from the realm of disgust, and placed in a cultural space of decency.

If the relatives of an Alzheimer's patient were to visit her in a nursing home and find her naked, eating from a dinner bowl like a dog, they might well describe what shocks them by saying, "They are treating her like an animal!" The shock is a response to her degraded condition, conceived in terms of a symbolic demotion to subhuman animal status. This shows that the ... dignity of humans is essentially tied to their human species membership, conceived hierarchically in relation to nonhuman animals and independently of the capacities of the individual whose dignity is at stake.[30]

When proponents of the AMC make the situation for those in 1 equivalent to the situation for those in 2, they are denying the very sensibility of this scenario.

How might the proponent of the AMC respond?

One response might simply be to say that humans with severe Alzheimer's, or those who are severely cognitively impaired, and non-human animals, who are not persons or moral agents, will command different sorts of treatment depending on the kinds of reasoned justifications that moral agents can make for that differential treatment and, as Anderson says, the types or relationships with moral patients those agents have. Nonetheless, there is no reason to invoke a hierarchy of moral status, where human moral patients are higher than non-human moral patients in virtue of their species-based connection to human moral agents. One can imagine that if one treated a dog like a horse, some human moral agent might object in a similar vein.[31] That the AMC equates the moral status of individuals in 1 with individuals in 2 does not mean that their treatment should now be identical or that there is nothing troubling or objectionable about treating a human like a dog, a dog like a horse, a chimpanzee like a human child.

In addition, consider the fact that different living options are available for parents with Alzheimer's. Adult children will often go to great lengths

---

[30] Ibid.: 282.

[31] Some object to greyhound racing on just these grounds, but I have in mind people riding on dogs.

to see that their ailing parents get the very best possible care, perhaps quite expensive care, even when their parent is completely unaware that they are being cared for in such an elaborate way. It is not for the parent's sake that this care is offered, but for the sake of the family and their peace of mind. Some families don't care for their ailing parents in these ways – because they can't afford such care; because they would rather spend what funds they have on the members of the family who are persons and can directly appreciate the benefit from such funds; or because they don't see it as their moral responsibility (perhaps the parent was abusive to the children who are now estranged from her). We don't force families to provide top-of-the-line care for their parents who are not persons. (Indeed, we don't have moral expectations that families provide top-of-the-line care for members who are persons.) A decent society would surely care for these individuals in ways that attend to their basic needs. The specific social relations will determine how moral agents come to understand their moral obligations to moral patients. A family who has their mother with Alzheimer's in a top-of-the-line facility might find the state-run care "undignified"; they might even think that the state-run facility "treats people like animals." But this judgment could be the result of snobbery or speciesism, and we should not draw moral conclusions from such judgments. These judgments, in themselves, don't show that human non-persons, by virtue of their social relations with other, sometimes judgmental, persons are due more consideration than non-human non-persons.

Kittay has also argued against the AMC on similar grounds. As the mother of a severely cognitively impaired daughter, named Sesha, Kittay is vividly attuned to the role of social relations in understanding our moral commitments to others. When we think of the individuals in 1, she wants us always to think of them as "someone's child . . . That social relationship [entails] a series of appropriate emotional and moral responses . . . It is morally (and emotionally) appropriate to care for one's child for the child's own sake. It is the practices that define parenthood, and not simply the intrinsic properties of the product of the pregnancy."[32] The intrinsic properties account leads to the conclusion that we may disregard individuals like Sesha and accept "treating her like an animal" just as consistently as it would require greater moral attention for people like Sesha and other animals. Kittay argues that we can avoid this risk by rejecting the intrinsic properties account for determining

---

[32] Kittay 2009: 145.

who belongs in what category and, instead, focusing on species-specific social relations that model the family. She writes:

> Family membership is conditional on birth lines, marriage, and (under particular conditions) adoption, not on having certain intrinsic properties ... Families (or adequate substitutes) are critical when we are dependent, as in early childhood, during acute or chronic illness, with serious chronic conditions including disability, and in frail old age. At these times, we are generally best served by close personal ties. Families are called on in times of moral crisis for the support of family love and loyalty. Similarly, I propose that membership in a group of moral peers based solely on species membership has as its appropriate moral analogue family membership, not racism ... As humans we are indeed a family.[33]

Here, Kittay is suggesting that partiality to one's own group, the "in" group, needn't be thought of as necessarily prejudicial. She is urging us to think of speciesism – favoring one's own species over members of other species – as on par with favoring one's own family. Insofar as we think it is ethically permissible to grant greater weight to the interests and desires of members of our own family, so is it permissible to grant greater weight to the interests and desires of members of our own species. Kittay is essentially denying premise 4 of the AMC.

There are a number of possible responses to this view. It might be suggested that ultimately we aren't morally justified in caring more about our own children and family members than the children and family members of our neighbors and colleagues; it is just a function of the way we have arranged our social relations and institutions that we are psychologically oriented toward favoring our own family members and, practically, it works out well if every family takes care of their own. There are, in fact, different cultural practices and alternative family arrangements in which caring for one's own family members more than for other people is not thought to be justifiable. Favoring one's own family and how we understand who counts as a family member are arguably artifacts of our particular social and cultural practices. And cultural practices are often the very sorts of practices that should be held up to ethical interrogation, because they tend to make certain kinds of prejudices seem natural, as I noted earlier. Even within our own culture, there are limits beyond which favoring one's own family members become questionable. We cannot go to any lengths to further the interests of our own children over the interests of other people's children. It would be quite objectionable, for example, if you were driving your child and a neighbor's child to school, for you to use both seatbelts to double-strap your child in while leaving your neighbor's child without a seatbelt. In addition to being limited, partiality to one's own family members is not thought to be ethically required. We don't think that the parent who sends her children to public school and sends the money she would have spent sending them to private school to support education in the developing world is doing something unethical; indeed, many would find that admirable. So, partiality to family looks more like a contingent feature of our social relations and not a principle for organizing our ethical obligations.

Families come in many forms. These days, families often include children from other marriages and various genetic parents, adopted children, the children of adopted children, girlfriends or boyfriends who have been rejected by their families of birth, orphaned cousins, etc. One might also argue that it is possible to think of "families" as including more than just humans. Many people have come to identify other animals as part of their family or intimate social units. Donna Haraway has written expansively about "companion species" who are not simply "pets" but other beings with whom we are in significant, life-altering relationships. She describes her own transformation as a result of working with her dog. Haraway says, "my over-the-top love for Cayenne has required my body to build a bigger heart with more depths and tones for tenderness. Maybe that is what makes me need to be honest; maybe this kind of love makes one need to see what is really happening because the loved one deserves it. There is nothing like the unconditional love that people ascribe to their dogs!"[34] George Pitcher describes the relationship he and his partner had with their two adopted dogs in distinctly familiar terms. He describes:

> their complete and unwavering devotion to us. They showed this constantly, in countless ways...We loved them with all our hearts...and they loved us, too, completely, no holds barred. Such love is perhaps the best thing life has to offer, and we shall always be grateful for having had such an abundance of it to receive and to give for so long a time...They were our surrogate children...Naturally the love of one's dog cannot be as deep and rich as the

[34] Haraway 2008: 215.

love of one's child, but it can be in some ways just as intense. For example, our concern for the welfare of Lupa and Remus was, I believe, as strong as a devoted father's for his child's.[35]

Dawn Prince-Hughes, an autistic writer and anthropologist, found the most comfort in the company of animals, and it was through her observations of, and work with, gorillas that she was eventually able to enter into a human family. Prince-Hughes, by spending time watching captive gorillas who were "so sensitive and so trapped," began to understand herself, the world, and other humans. Through them she learned that "persons are more than chaotic knots of random actions" and "that as people we are reflected in one another. Because the gorillas were so like me in so many ways, I was able to see myself in them, and in turn, I saw them – and eventually myself – in other human people."[36] Bonds of kinship extend beyond the species border, in our own culture and in others. If other animals can be part of families, then the family does not serve as a model for identifying morally relevant distinctions between species.

Taking offense

Kittay has simply denied the possibility that other animals can be members of our families in the relevant way; indeed, she finds the idea offensive. She has lived with and loved dogs, but to compare her feelings for her dog with those for her daughter is, it seems, unthinkable for her. She writes:

> How can I begin to tell you what it feels like to read texts in which one's child is compared, in all seriousness and with philosophical authority, to a dog, pig, rat, and most flatteringly a chimp; how corrosive these comparisons are, how they mock those relationships that affirm who we are and why we care? I am no stranger to a beloved animal. I have had dogs I have loved, dogs I have mourned for. But as dog lovers who become parents can tell you, much as we adore our hounds, there is no comparison between the feelings for a beloved child of normal capacities and those for a beloved canine. And I can tell you that there is also no comparison when that child has intellectual disabilities.[37]

---

[35] Pitcher 1995: 158–9, 162, and 163, as quoted in McMahan 2005: 364.
[36] Prince-Hughes 2004: 3.   [37] Kittay 2009: 610.

The comparisons between severely cognitively impaired humans, like Sesha, with non-human moral patients are not just unthinkable but sickening. Kittay continues:

> to articulate the differences between a human animal with significantly curtailed cognitive capacities and a relatively intelligent nonhuman animal means that one first has to see the former as the latter. That is the moment of revulsion . . . Note that this response has little to do with the affection one might feel for a nonhuman animal . . . Imagine, if you can, taking the person that you love as much as you love anything in this world, your beloved child, and looking at her with the comparative measure of a dog or a rat or a chimp or a pig . . . what makes this particular case so toxic is that the relentless comparisons of my daughter to a nonhuman animal, this dehumanization, is in itself the objectification of her.[38]

A person's experience of emotional distress over a philosophical argument is certainly something to take note of, and the distress and frustration that Kittay feels when presented with the AMC should not simply be dismissed. But that one is offended is not enough to disprove an argument, nor is it enough to justify, without further examination, certain questionable practices. Consider the fact that many pious men are repulsed and offended by the sight of a woman who is not completely covered in a burqa. Many racists are disgusted when they encounter black people in positions of power. These feelings can lead to ethically objectionable practices. As we have just discussed, our feelings may be the result of certain cultural or traditional assumptions that themselves do not hold up to critical ethical scrutiny. In addition, some parents of severely cognitively impaired children may find the comparisons between 1 and 2 in the AMC offensive and others may not. Some people have an expansive capacity for love: they can love their children, each one differently but fully, and they can love the animals with whom they share their lives.[39] Some parents have come to deeply love particular animals when they see it is with those animals that their severely cognitively impaired children are their happiest and most comforted. Feelings about family members vary from culture to culture and between individuals within cultures. Feelings of

---

[38] Ibid.: 613.

[39] As Mary Midgley 1983: 119 puts it: "One sort of love does not need to block another, because love, like compassion, is not a rare fluid to be economized, but a capacity which grows by use."

revulsion, disgust, and horror at arguments may be an indication that an argument should be explored more carefully, but such feelings, alone, can't refute an argument.

Just as a parent of a severely cognitively disabled child may be disgusted by the comparison of her child with non-human animals, some people who work with animals find the comparison of normally functioning adult animals with cognitively impaired humans offensive. If we think back to the hippopotamus at the beginning of this chapter, we see an individual who is independent, can take care of her own needs, acts intentionally, coexists with others relatively peacefully, defends the weak, and apparently tries to help the injured. The dolphins, chimpanzees, and birds we have discussed all engage in complex social and cognitively sophisticated behaviors. These non-human animals are capable of doing things that are sometimes far beyond the abilities of human individuals with severe cognitive deficits who are unable to clothe themselves, feed themselves, clean themselves, or perhaps even recognize others.

Those who worry about the sensibility of equating normal non-humans with cognitively deficient humans might ask where non-humans with cognitive impairments fit in. Other animals too suffer from cognitive disability. I know a chimpanzee named Knuckles who has cognitive and motor-control deficits believed to be due to cerebral palsy. Knuckles has lived at a sanctuary called the Center for Great Apes since he was two years old, and there he receives round-the-clock care from human caregivers, while also being allowed supervised visits with other chimpanzees. Due to the diligent care of the sanctuary staff and volunteers, Knuckles has learned to feed himself, climb up and down steps, and pull himself up on special swings to hang upside down and play. He is aware of activities around him, likes to play with other chimpanzees, and is very affectionate. He is, however, quite distinct in his abilities from other non-cognitively impaired chimpanzees, who are also quite distinct from humans with cognitive impairments.

The point of the comparison of those in 1 with those in 2 of the AMC is not to diminish either but to point to an inconsistency in our attitudes and behaviors toward moral patients. When proponents of the AMC argue that humans with severe cognitive impairments are not persons, just as many non-human animals are not persons, they are not "demoting" the humans to the status of animals. We are all animals. Rather, they are attempting to rectify a mischaracterization of the moral universe that is based on species prejudice. All moral patients, human or non-human, cognitively able or cognitively impaired, have interests that deserve our moral attention. But that does not ensure that their interests will always win out when there are conflicts of interests, just as is the case when conflicts between persons occur and everyone's interests cannot be simultaneously satisfied. Greater knowledge of the specific kinds of interests that different moral patients have will enhance our abilities to resolve conflicts in the most ethically defensible ways. Kittay and others who have personal stakes in the lives of human non-persons have succeeded in making more vivid the importance and value of the lives, experiences, and interests of those living with severe cognitive abilities, and have reminded us of the importance of epistemic humility. But there is no reason to extend that humility to all humans then stop at the species border. Those studying and caring for non-human animals have also enlivened our understanding of the value of the lives, experiences, and interests of other animals. Comparing the two is only offensive if one assumes that the lives of other animals are less valuable or worthy of our attention, and, as I have been arguing, that assumption is based on an unjustifiable prejudice.

The natural world contains hippopotamuses and crocodiles, dandelions and dugongs, philosophers and biologists, Sesha and Knuckles. The categories we now use to distinguish between these various organisms are not something that we can read off the natural world; we need to make distinctions and judgments about how to categorize, and then give meaning to those categories. This is where the normative enters. Whether we tie our normative evaluations to individual natural properties or relations between organisms and their environments, or both, those who can make judgments, what I have been calling persons, have certain ethical and epistemological responsibilities, including justifying the value placed on the various categories as constructed and, perhaps most importantly, being able to defend that valuation in light of the implication these value commitments have in practice. It is to the practices that we will now turn.

3   Eating animals

It has often been said that if people were required to kill the animals they eat, they would become vegetarians. In one year, a household of four people in the United States eats approximately three-quarters of a cow, one and a third pigs, seventy chickens, and four turkeys. If they were to kill all these animals themselves, they would be slaughtering animals at least once a week (and would need a very large freezer). But it isn't only the use of time and space that might put people off eating other animals. The repulsion would come from having to look into an animal's eyes while yielding a knife and slitting her throat.

Most people don't have the time, space, or temperament to slaughter other animals to eat them, and they don't have to because large intensive slaughterhouses and processing plants exist to do the job for them. In the United States alone, these massive industrialized operations are capable of slaughtering and processing about ten billion animals annually, and the killing is designed to be swift and mechanical. In a single chicken slaughterhouse, for example, the birds are killed at a rate averaging 7,500 an hour, about two birds per second. The process involves shackling birds upside down by their feet from an overhead conveyor belt, dipping their heads into an electrified water tank to stun them, and then whizzing them past a sharp revolving blade that slices their necks. They are then dropped into a scalding tank that prepares their carcasses for de-feathering and dismemberment. The chickens are moving so fast, often only shackled by one leg, that when they aren't sufficiently stunned, they struggle to free themselves. That struggle can cause the killing blade to cut through only part of their necks, and if the human "killer" on the floor at the time misses the kill, the chicken ends up boiled alive.

One such "killer," the late Virgil Butler, described his experiences working at Tyson Foods' Grannis, Arkansas processing plant. Tyson Foods is the world's largest food-processing company and processes an estimated 2 billion chickens each year.

The killing machine can never slit the throat of every bird that goes by, especially those that the stunner does not stun properly. So, you have what is known as a "killer" whose job it is to catch those birds so that they are not scalded alive in the tank....

No matter what the weather is like outside, this room is hot, between 90–100F. The scalders also keep the humidity at about 100%. You can see the steam in the air as a kind of haze. You put on your plastic apron to cover your whole body from the sprays of blood and the hot water that keeps the killing machine's blade clean and washes the floor. You put on the steel glove and pick up the knife. It's very sharp. It has to be.

You can hear the squawking from the chickens being hung in the next room as well as the metal shackles rattling. Here come the birds through the stunner into the killing machine. You can expect to have to catch every 5th one or so, many that are not stunned. They come at you 182–186 per minute. There is blood everywhere, in the $3' \times 3' \times 20'$ trough beneath the machine, on your face, your neck, your arms, all down your apron. You are covered in it. Sometimes you have to wash off the clots of blood, without taking your eyes off the line lest one slip by....

You can't catch them all, but you try. You see it flopping around in the scalder, beating itself against the sides ... another "redbird." You know that for every one you see suffer like this, there have been as many as 10 you didn't see.

The sheer amount of killing and blood can really get to you after a while, especially if you can't just shut down all emotion completely ... You feel like part of a big death machine. Pretty much treated that way as well. Sometimes weird thoughts will enter your head. It's just you and the dying chickens. The surreal feelings grow into such a horror of the barbaric nature of your behavior.

You are murdering helpless birds by the thousands (75,000 to 90,000 a night).

You are a killer

You shut down all emotions eventually. You just can't care about anything. Because if you care about something, it opens the gate to all those bad feelings that you can't afford to feel and still do your job. You have bills to pay. You have to eat.

But, you don't want chicken. You have to be really hungry to eat that.[1]

---

[1] From the CyberActivist, "Inside the Mind of a Killer" http://cyberactivist.blogspot.com/2003/08/inside-mind-of-killer.html.

Butler, a self-described hillbilly from rural Arkansas, started out in the chicken industry as a "catcher" when he was a teenager. He would travel to various contract farms for Tyson, go into the chicken houses, grab the chickens, and stuff them into crates to be transported to slaughterhouses. Later he got a steady job killing chickens at Tyson plants. He worked killing chickens for five years before he could no longer do the job. It was certainly hard work, but, apparently, what got to Virgil was his inability to accept the suffering he was causing and admit what he did for a living to his loved ones. Even though he was raised to believe "they are just damned chickens," over time their blood and terror were too much for him. He ended up getting fired from Tyson in 2002 after missing work repeatedly, became a vegetarian, and, until his death in December 2006, worked tirelessly to expose what was happening on America's factory farms.

The scenes that Butler recounts are not so different from those Upton Sinclair described a century earlier in *The Jungle*, his graphic exposé of abuses of workers and animals occurring in Chicago's unregulated slaughterhouses. While methods for transporting, slaughtering, and processing animals have not changed in meaningful ways for the animals, one thing certainly has changed – the methods of rearing animals before they are transported to meet their ends. In the early 1900s, most animals were raised on small, independent farms and ranches, where the ranchers and farmers and their families had direct relationships with the animals. Knowledge about how to care for the animals was passed down from previous generations, and stories about the quirks and antics of the animals were shared at the end of long working days. Animals were typically outdoors, relatively free to move around, and able to socialize with others of their kind. They were protected from predators and had fairly pleasant lives. All that began to change in the 1920s, as farming became more industrialized.

The evolution of industrial agriculture

In the 1900s, there were over six million farms throughout the US. A century later, there were approximately two million farms, and the size of each was roughly triple that of the farms of old. This trend toward a smaller number of much larger operations is the direct result of the industrialization of agriculture. In 1926, the US Secretary of Agriculture encouraged the transformation of farms into factories, stating: "The United States has become great industrially largely through mass production which facilitates elimination of waste and lowering of overhead costs ... tremendous economies both in production and distribution has [*sic*] enabled manufacturers to supply consumers with what they want when they want it. It seems to me that in this matter agriculture must follow the example of industry."[2] Of course, not all of these farms were dedicated to raising animals, but those that were faced unique challenges, not the least of which was figuring out how to keep a large number of animals alive in a confined space.

Chickens were the first to be transformed into mass-produced commodities, although they were not sent directly to factory farms but rather to laboratories in agricultural colleges across the country where "animal husbandry" became "animal science." As the Republican party of the 1920s was campaigning on the slogan "a chicken in every pot," poultry scientists were studying chicken reproduction, health, and nutrition in order to figure out a way to rear chickens intensively. Of all animals raised for food, chickens proved to be relatively good laboratory subjects. They had short lifespans and were small enough to be caged, and their early development could be studied outside of their mothers' bodies, in eggs. Still it was not easy to keep the birds confined their entire lives. Initially, the lack of ultraviolet light contributed to a nutritional deficiency that created leg weakness.[3] Adding Vitamin D to chicken feed allowed scientists, and ultimately farmers, to overcome this particular difficulty for intensive confinement. But as chickens were being confined in greater numbers, additional problems emerged, particularly problems with contagious diseases. If one chicken became sick, it would not be long before the whole flock, now confined in tight quarters, would become sick. In the 1940s, antibiotic use was introduced into industrialized animal farming, and it fundamentally changed the industry. In addition to helping control the spread of disease, adding antibiotics to feed increased the weight of chickens by 10 percent or more, and it turned out that antibiotics had a growth-promoting effect on other animals as well.[4] In 1954, 2 million pounds of antibiotics were produced in the United States, and roughly a quarter of this supply was used in livestock feed. Within ten years, the amount of antibiotics used more than doubled, and by the late 1990s, over 25 million pounds of antibiotics were fed to animals on industrial farms in the US. As we will see later in this chapter, the regular use of antibiotics and

---

[2] As cited in Fitzgerald 2003: 108.   [3] Boyd 2001.   [4] Ibid.: 647.

antimicrobials in animal agriculture has had worrisome consequences on public health.

Adding antibiotics to animal feed is just one of the ways that industrialized farmers were able to increase the growth of animals. Manipulating their genomes, both through trial-and-error breeding and, more recently, through laboratory interventions to genetically modify animals, has allowed for faster development of larger, "meatier" animals in less time. Again, this all started with chickens, or, more precisely, with eggs. The older breeds of chicken initially bred for slaughter required seventy to eighty days to grow to their final weight of just under three pounds, and the "feed conversion ratio" – that is, the number of pounds of food it takes to produce a pound of chicken – was four to one. Today, chickens reach an average slaughter weight of about five pounds in only forty-five days, and the feed conversion ratio is now less than two to one.[5]

The ability to grow larger animals, in less time and for less direct cost, could only have occurred when companies were large enough to exert control over all aspects of the industry – from production through marketing – so as to make profits more predictable, which, in turn, allowed for more investment in research. Tyson Foods, Inc. is a prime example of a corporation that not only controls production, but also influences the marketplace, even creating products that consumers didn't know they wanted. From its humble beginnings in spring 1936, when John W. Tyson, a small-time Arkansas trucker, drove 500 chickens to sell to the big Chicago slaughterhouses, Tyson Foods, Inc. has become the "the largest provider of protein products on the planet," achieved primarily through a process known as "vertical integration." Tyson Foods owns all the hatcheries, feed mills, and slaughter and processing plants it uses to produce animals. And the top ten integrated firms now control over 75 percent of chicken production in the US, so they influence the market as well. They contract out the process of growing chickens to smaller operations, but the companies maintain ownership of the chickens. Although sometimes referred to as "family farmers," these smaller "grow-out" operations don't look anything like the family farms of old. Integrators often require growers to maintain expensive state-of-the-art chicken houses in which up to 30,000 birds are crammed and monitored by high-tech equipment. Computers give growers up-to-the-second reports on temperature, feeding and watering

[5] Barrett 2002b. See also Tyson Foods, Inc. 2008.

systems output, and chicken weight. Heaters, coolers, lights, humidifiers, and ventilation are automated and respond to computer outputs. These high-end modern chicken houses can cost between $175,000 and $200,000 each. While this automation may seem to make things easier for the contract grower, the debt they bear makes these small growers vulnerable to the changing whims of the integrators. Growers must accept the terms of the contracts in order to make ends meet. In addition, as one contract grower put it, "you become a prisoner to your farm . . . I've got pagers that alert me when something's wrong but you only have a few minutes to react. In the past, when the houses weren't so dependent on technology, you had more time to adjust the temperature or the water. Now, you've got to get there quick or else you'll lose thousands of birds."[6]

In addition to vertical integration, the large corporations have diversified – they don't simply grow and slaughter one type of animal, but are involved in turning a variety of animals into consumer products. Tyson Foods, Inc. is the largest cow slaughterer and the second largest pig slaughterer in the US.[7] In 2008, on average, they killed 40 million chickens, 141,860 cows, and 393,350 pigs *per week*.[8] One of their "fun facts" states that they sell "enough chicken tenderloins in one year that if you placed them end to end, they would circle the earth 3.7 times." And it isn't just their imagined chicken tenderloins traversing the earth, but the actual body parts of all sorts of animals raised, processed, and sold around the world.

Globally, an estimated 53 billion animals are killed for consumption each year. Worldwide consumption of animals has increased more than fivefold since 1950, and factory farms, or what government agencies and the industry are now referring to as CAFOs – concentrated animal feeding operations – are being set up in many countries, particularly those that have relatively lax regulations and enforcement.[9] Tyson Foods, Inc. also has processing plants in Argentina, Brazil, China, India, Indonesia, Japan, Mexico, the Netherlands, the Philippines, Russia, Spain, the United Kingdom, and Venezuela. Tyson's annual sales for 2008 were $26.9 billion. Their next largest competitor, multinational Smithfield Foods, the largest producer of pigs globally, reported almost $12.5 billion in annual sales for 2009.[10] Smithfield Foods has also

---

[6] Barrett 2002b.   [7] Hendrickson & Heffernan 2007.   [8] Tyson Foods, Inc. 2008.
[9] The relatively new CAFO terminology is potentially misleading as there is much more that happens on factory farms than animal feeding.
[10] Smithfield Foods 2009.

expanded their factory farming operations globally over the last decade. They opened facilities in Romania, one of the poorest countries in the European Union, and, in the process, by mass-producing pigs, were able to lower prices temporarily, thus forcing roughly 90 percent of the small, family farms out of business in just a four-year period.[11] Many of the local farmers sold their land and left the country to look for work.

Factory farms do more than destroy livelihoods, they can also damage the quality of life in the communities in which they are located. In 2005 *The Chicago Tribune* reported that in Poland, where Smithfield has also expanded, a Smithfield subsidiary was operating a large pig factory farm in the town of Wieckowice. The report claimed that the waste from the pigs was being disposed of near the local school, causing students to vomit and faint. The company changed the location of the waste to the other end of its property, closer to a lake, but then local residents complained that the water smelled odd and that their children who swam in the lake were developing eye infections.[12]

While the quality of life for people living near factory farms is degraded by their presence, life for animals on factory farms is devoid of all quality. Their lives are full of pain, fear, and frustration until they are slaughtered.

Living and dying on factory farms

In a technological trade magazine article extolling the virtues of high-tech industrial animal production, the journey of one Tyson chicken, from birth to death, is told from his point of view. It reads:

> It all started nearly 50 days ago when I poked my egg tooth out of my shell. In just a couple of hours, I was on a truck from the hatchery to the grow-out farm where I would spend the next 46 days of my life. At the farm, I was quickly unloaded and put into a house with about 20,000 other chicks.... For the first five days, the lights were kept on around the clock. There was nothing else to do but eat, drink and answer the call of nature, so when the lights were on we did lots of eating... On and after the 26th day, we were basically kept in the dark.... After a while, the house became a bit stuffy and started to smell.... Day 47 began as the previous 21 had but something different happened. Suddenly the door to the house was opened and we were

[11] Carvajal & Castle 2009.   [12] Hundley 2005.

awkwardly herded and – in most cases – tossed into the back of a large truck.... After about a 75-mile drive, we arrived at the processing plant. This would be one of the few times that a human being actually put his hands on us. They grabbed us by our legs and hung us upside down ... Think of it as an assembly line toward dismemberment ...

My breasts have been halved, breaded and shipped to their current resting-place on a shelf in a supermarket in Denver. My legs should be arriving in Moscow any time now. All my feathers have been processed and are now being eaten by cattle somewhere in Texas. My blood and bones have been rendered for cat food, fertilizer and who-knows-what else. My wings have been seasoned with barbecue sauce and served with a side of ranch dressing and celery at some bar and grill in New York City. My feet? Well, they're headed to Asia where I'm told they're something of a delicacy.[13]

While there is much that is striking about this little tale, what is perhaps most telling is that the story contains no mention of the suffering most commonly experienced on factory farms, not just by chickens and hens, but by pigs, sows, cows, cattle, and the other animals who live and die in industrial agriculture.

Chickens

In addition to the billions of chickens who are killed globally, there are an estimated five billion laying hens in the world, each producing roughly 300 eggs per year. Most of these hens are kept in small wire cages, called "battery cages," with between three and eight other hens. The battery cages are stacked on top of each other indoors in sheds that can contain upward of 100,000 hens. The battery cage is so small that the hens are unable to stretch their wings or turn around. Because of the stress, boredom, fear, and close quarters, hens will peck at each other, so most are routinely debeaked, a process that involves a hot blade cutting off the tip of the beak through a thick layer of highly sensitive tissue. Debeaking causes lasting pain and impairs the hen's ability to eat, drink, wipe her beak, and preen normally.

Because eating eggs doesn't require killing the hen, many think that eating eggs is ethically acceptable or at least better than eating chickens and other animals. This is usually not the case. Life as a battery hen is one of the worst lives endured by any animal in industrial agriculture, except perhaps that of sows in large hog operations. Chickens living in naturalistic environments

---

[13] Barrett 2002a.

can live up to ten years, but in battery operations, they are killed after just one. They begin laying when they are between eighteen and twenty weeks old, and sometimes they are starved and forced to molt in order to prolong production. But, when their productivity inevitably declines, they are considered "spent hens" and sent to slaughter.

In natural conditions, chickens live in stable social groups of around thirty birds. They establish social hierarchies and can recognize where each bird is in "the pecking order." They typically use their beaks to manipulate their environments and to forage for food. Hens always nest, and they form strong ties to their chicks, bonding with them even before they hatch by turning the eggs while clucking. Once a hen's chicks hatch, she will watch over them as one would expect from a "mother hen." Chickens are intelligent and communicative, and they have been observed courageously defending their young from predators – not the stereotypical view of a chicken. These typical behaviors are completely frustrated in industrial chicken and egg production.

Pigs

The lives of female animals on factory farms are particularly difficult. Hens, sows, and cows are forced to live under cruel conditions for longer than their male counterparts as their reproductive capacities are exploited to extract as much profitable product as possible. Breeding sows are kept indoors in gestation crates throughout most of their adult lives. These barren stalls fit tightly around the sow, and she is unable to turn around and can only stand and then lie down again with difficulty. The sows are denied virtually all social interaction and are unable to engage in any species-typical behaviors. Pigs are highly social animals who ordinarily would live in small, matriarchal groups. When living in more naturalistic environments, pigs interact regularly with one another, huddling and grooming together. They have distinct personalities and develop specific relationships with others of their kind. Their social and tactile interactions are a central part of their daily lives in natural settings, but on factory farms they are denied any opportunity to interact. Even when a sow gives birth, she is given virtually no access to her piglets; they can suck up to her teats, but she cannot move to help them or nuzzle them. A sow ordinarily builds nests before giving birth to provide herself and her piglets a soft place to lie down, but even this basic instinct is frustrated. In two to four weeks, her piglets are taken from her to be fattened up for market, and she is usually impregnated again. A typical breeding sow will have six to seven pregnancies in three to four years before she is sent to slaughter.

After being abruptly taken from their mother, piglets are kept indoors in barren, overcrowded pens, sometimes in cages stacked on top of one another. While pigs are not ordinarily aggressive, under stress they can be, and pigs in intensive rearing conditions are known to bite others' tails. Rather than provide more space, and minimize stress, factory farmers will have pigs' tails docked and teeth clipped to prevent tail biting.

Recent studies suggest that pigs have a high degree of intelligence and social cognition, not unlike elephants, dolphins, and great apes, which makes them unique among domesticated animals. They have been shown to be able to recognize mirrors and use reflected images to solve environmental problems, a skill indicative of high levels of cognition.[14] Denying pigs every possibility of expressing their intelligence through extreme confinement causes them great stress. In addition, their confinement causes them to suffer chronic physical pain due to reduced muscle tone and bone strength. With no outlet for their frustration, many pigs exhibit abnormal stereotypies, including pacing, bar biting, and vacuum chewing (chewing when nothing is present). Perhaps it is a blessing that their frustrating lives are short. Pigs are fattened up for six months and then sent to slaughter. Wild pigs can live more than fifteen years.

Cows

Like sows, dairy cows' bodies endure enormous demands. The global estimate for milk production is 166,850 million gallons annually. Over 200 million dairy cows produce this milk at great physiological costs. They are often producing more milk than the calories they have taken in and will begin to metabolize their own muscle in order to continue to produce milk, a process referred to in the industry as "milking off their back." Cows are milked by machines and often suffer from painful inflammation of the mammary glands, or mastitis. Intensive confinement, over-production of milk, and constant pregnancies also put cows at great risk for other painful infectious diseases. Dairy cows produce milk for approximately ten months after giving

[14] Watson 2004 and Broom, et al. 2009.

birth. They are kept in a cycle of pregnancy and lactation for three to seven years until they are considered "spent," at which point they are slaughtered.

Calves are separated from their mothers within twenty-four hours; the females are usually kept to replace their mothers as milk producers, and the males are sent to be fattened up and slaughtered. Some of the male calves will be sent off to become veal. The veal industry is a direct outgrowth of the dairy industry. With a surplus of unwanted male calves, there was profit to be made in the creation of a "delicacy" of tender meat that "melts in one's mouth." In order to create flesh of this consistency, calves are chained by the neck in wooden crates so that they are unable to move. Movement would strengthen their muscles, creating tougher flesh. The calves are fed a liquid diet, deficient in iron and fiber, designed to keep their flesh light in color. This deprivation goes on for eighteen to twenty weeks, and then the calves are slaughtered.

The suffering that animals endure in industrialized agriculture is extreme. As we discussed in the previous chapters, practices in which an individual's interests are ignored, practices that involve forcing others to experience pain and deprivation, and practices that deny individuals the respect they are due require ethical justification. Under most circumstances, humans do not need to consume animals in order to survive. Most of us have access to nutritious food that does not involve causing animals to live and die in horrible conditions. It seems that the only justification for causing other animals such harm through factory farming is the satisfaction of the human desire to eat animals, and that is no justification at all.

Arguments against factory farms

Conditions on factory farms should cause everyone to pause before purchasing meat products and contributing to the lifetime of pain, terror, and anguish other animals endure in industrial agriculture. By purchasing industrial animal products, consumers are directly contributing to, and indirectly condoning, the practices that cause so much suffering to other sensitive animals. Most of the time, the pleasure derived from eating animals' bodies in no way outweighs the lives of pain those animals endured. That so many animals suffer so greatly should be reason enough to start eliminating industrial animal production. Yet there are additional reasons to end the practice. In this section, we will look briefly at other reasons why we should condemn factory farming, for the sake of all animals, humans and others, as well as for the sake of the planet that sustains us all.

Environmental destruction

Throughout the US and across the world, factory farms are creating all sorts of environmental problems. CAFOs confine large numbers of animals in small spaces. (To be officially classified as a CAFO, an individual facility must contain at least 1,000 cows, 2,500 pigs, or 125,000 chickens.) As the number of animals raised on CAFOs increases, the amount of animal waste produced increases, too. However, the capacity of the land to absorb that waste does not suddenly increase as well. These facilities generate huge amounts of urine and excrement, which is liquefied and stored either under the buildings where the animals live or in nearby open-pit lagoons. The US Department of Agriculture (USDA) estimates that in the US livestock and poultry produce 335 million tons of manure per year. In Iowa alone, hogs excrete 50 million tons of manure annually. Overall, animals excrete forty times as much fecal waste as humans do.[15] All this waste releases high levels of ammonia and hydrogen sulfide (a gas that smells like rotten eggs). The breakdown of organic carbon and nitrogen compounds in manure leads to the emission of noxious levels of gases. Chicken producers in the top ten chicken-producing states released an estimated 481 million pounds of ammonia in 2007, or more than eight times the combined total reported by industrial sources.[16]

In addition to polluting the air, CAFOs are a major source of water pollution. While manure was once spread on the land as fertilizer, the ground in most areas has now reached saturation. In the Chesapeake Bay area, for example, poultry manure is the largest source of excess nitrogen and phosphorus reaching the Chesapeake from the lower Eastern Shore, and these two nutrients, in excess, overstimulate algae growth. When algae die, their decomposition consumes oxygen, choking fish and other water life. Well water is also contaminated. According to a study by the US Geological Survey (USGS), as many as one-third of all wells in the Chesapeake Bay area exceed US Environmental Protection Agency (EPA) safe drinking-water standards for nitrate, a form of nitrogen concentrated in chicken waste that seeps into groundwater. The USGS also found trace amounts of arsenic, the likely residue of

[15] Bittman 2008.   [16] Environmental Integrity Project 2008.

arsenic added to chicken feed to kill harmful parasites and promote growth. And there are other ways that chicken waste pollutes the water. Every day, chicken slaughterhouses along the lower Eastern Shore kill more than 2 million birds and use more than 12 million gallons of water to flush away more than 3 million pounds of guts, chicken heads, feathers, and blood.[17] The water-pollution problem is not localized to the Chesapeake Bay area, of course, and it isn't limited to industrial chicken production. An EPA official in charge of water reported on the spill of pig waste in North Carolina. An eight-acre lagoon of waste "burst through its dike, spilling approximately 22 million gallons of animal waste into the New River. The spill was twice the size of the Exxon Valdez oil spill." This official testified that "animal operations, including feedlots and animal holding areas, affect 20% of impaired river miles, or about 35,000 river miles in these 22 States."[18] According to the USDA, "animal waste in the United States has been estimated to contribute about 50 percent of all anthropogenic ammonia emissions, 25 percent of nitrous oxide emissions, and 18 percent of methane emissions."[19] And in developing and emerging countries the "livestock sector" is the leading source of water pollution.[20]

Perhaps the most troubling environmental consequence of intensive animal production is its impact on global climate change. The UN Food and Agriculture report, *Livestock's Long Shadow*, claims that between 14 percent and 22 percent of the 36 billion tons of "CO_2-equivalent" greenhouse gases produced in the world every year is the result of animal production. Globally, "the livestock sector" emits more greenhouse gases than all forms of transportation combined. Cows emit between 2.5 and 4.7 ounces of methane for each pound of beef their bodies produce, and methane has approximately twenty-three times the global-warming potential of CO_2.[21] Some are arguing that because methane breaks down relatively quickly this estimate does not fully account for the dire impact methane emissions have on global warming. If the time horizon is shortened and the impact of methane is estimated over the next twenty years, it becomes seventy-two times more potent than CO_2.

Estimates over the next century are very serious – cows on CAFOs will produce thirty-six times more greenhouse gas emissions than are emitted by producing asparagus and twenty-four times more CO_2 than the nutritionally

[17] Goodman 1999.   [18] Cook 1998.   [19] USDA 2008.
[20] Steinfeld, et al. 2006: 267.   [21] Fiala 2009.

equivalent serving of rice and vegetables.[22] If the time horizon is shortened, then it appears that animal agriculture becomes the most important source of greenhouse gas emissions in countries like Australia, Brazil, and the US. According to one account, "Australia's methane emissions come primarily from 28 million cattle, 88 million sheep and a bunch of leaky coal mines. The livestock emissions, on their own, will cause significantly more warming in the next 20 years than all the coal fired power stations."[23] The impact of "livestock" emissions is serious enough that Rajendra Pachauri, the chair of the Intergovernmental Panel on Climate Change (IPCC), made an explicit call urging individuals to "Please eat less meat – meat is a very carbon intensive commodity . . . This is something that the IPCC was afraid to say earlier, but now we have said it."[24] As concerns about global climate change have grown, many are trying to minimize their "carbon footprint," and one direct way to do this is to stop eating other animals.

Public health concerns

There is another aspect of industrial animal production raising concerns beyond the welfare of the animals and the damage to the environment – the risks that closely confined animals, who are fed nontherapeutic levels of antibiotics and antimicrobials, pose to human health. Public health researchers, like Ellen Silbergeld of Johns Hopkins Bloomberg School of Public Health, are convinced that nontherapeutic use of antimicrobials is building dangerous genetic reservoirs of resistance and that factory farms are fostering drug-resistant bacteria that impair medicine's ability to protect the public from them. Kellogg Schwab, director of the Johns Hopkins Center for Water and Health, sampled a typical pig farm manure lagoon and found "trillions of bacteria present, of which 89 percent are resistant to drugs." He admits that these drug-resistant bacteria "scare the hell" out of him. "If we lose the ability to fight these microorganisms, a robust, healthy individual has a chance of dying, where before we would be able to prevent that death." Schwab says that if he tried, he could not build a better incubator of resistant pathogens than a factory farm.[25]

Schwab's fears are well founded. The USDA's Animal and Plant Health Inspection Service conducted large-scale, voluntary surveys in 1999, 2001,

---

[22] Subak 1999.   [23] Russell, et al. 2008.   [24] Quoted ibid.   [25] Quoted in Keiger 2009.

and 2006 that revealed that 84 percent of pig farms, 83 percent of cattle feedlots, and 84 percent of sheep farms use antimicrobials in the feed or water to
promote growth, and many scientific studies confirm that the nontherapeutic use of antibiotics in agricultural animals contributes to the development
of antibiotic-resistant bacterial infections in people. The General Accounting Office found that resistant strains of three microorganisms that cause
food-borne illness or disease in humans – salmonella, campylobacter, and
E. coli – are linked to the use of antibiotics in animals; the Food and Drug
Administration's National Antimicrobial Resistance Monitoring System routinely finds that retail meat products are contaminated with bacteria resistant to antibiotics important in human medicine, including the food-borne
pathogens campylobacter and salmonella; and the USDA issued a fact sheet
on the recently recognized link between antimicrobial drug use in animals
and methicillin-resistant *Staphylococcus aureus* (MRSA) infections in humans.[26]

The Union of Concerned Scientists suggests that approximately 60 percent
to 80 percent of all antibiotics used in the US are fed to farm animals to
promote growth, and efforts are being taken to end the use of antimicrobials for nontherapeutic purposes.[27] Spokespeople for intensive agriculture
claim that such estimates are significantly overblown and resist efforts to
limit the use of antimicrobials. They suggest that worries about resistance
should not be focused on the use of antimicrobials in industrial animal
production. According to Kristina Butts, the manager of legislative affairs
for the National Cattlemen's Beef Association, "resistance is the result of
human use and not related to veterinary use."[28] Expressing concern about
the health risks associated with resistant pathogens, the American Medical
Association, in 2001, passed a resolution opposing the use of antimicrobials
at nontherapeutic levels in agriculture and urged the termination of nontherapeutic use, in animals, of antimicrobials used in humans. In 2006, the
European Union prohibited the use of all antibiotics used in human medicine
as growth promoters in animals. The United States Congress may soon do the
same.

We can acquire resistant bacteria when we eat animals that carry them and
do not use proper hygienic techniques during preparation. Farm workers are

[26] House of Representatives 2009. See also Department of Health and Human Services 2005.
www.cdc.gov/narms/faq_antiresis.htm and United States General Accounting Office 2004.
www.gao.gov/new.items/d04490.pdf.

[27] Mellon, et al. 2001.   [28] Walsh 2009.

also at risk of exposure to drug-resistant bacteria and can transfer resistant infections to the broader public if they become ill. And antibiotic-resistant bacteria can reach the human community through surface and groundwater that have been contaminated by farm animal waste. More severe illnesses result in both higher frequency and longer duration of hospitalizations, and many resistant strains of bacteria are acquired by patients during hospitalization. According to a 2008 study, in the US, approximately two million people have become infected at hospitals, and, of those, 90,000 have died because their infections were immune to treatment.[29]

While bacterial resistance is a genuine concern, the new strains of species-crossing viruses are, perhaps, a greater worry. This concern emerged most vividly in the recent "swine flu pandemic." Because pigs are genetically similar enough to humans, they are susceptible to human flu viruses. They are also susceptible to avian viruses and have been referred to as "mixing vessels," in which strains of human, avian, and swine influenza swap genetic material to become even more potent. These potent viruses can jump from pigs to humans and back again. Virologists have suggested that pigs were the intermediate hosts responsible for the birth of the last two flu pandemics, in 1957 and 1968, as well as the more recent influenza A (H1N1) virus (S-OIV).[30] Not surprisingly, large concentrations of pigs on factory farms increase the risk of human exposure to these viruses, because humans who work on factory farms come in contact with a large number of animals on a regular basis. The first known cases of the 2009 pandemic were reported in the village of La Gloria, near Perote in the Mexican state of Veracruz. Perote is home to Smithfield Foods subsidiary Granjas Carroll de México. Factory farms are increasingly viewed as incubators of disease, and governments, as well as health and consumer protection organizations, are beginning to realize that the way animals are raised on factory farms is linked directly to a negative impact on human health.

There are so many reasons for rejecting factory farming, from a variety of different practical and theoretical perspectives, that it is hard to imagine what ethical arguments might be mounted in defense of this method of converting other animals into food products. Indeed, most of the arguments that are raised in support of factory farming are not really ethical arguments, but rather economic arguments with ethical implications.

---

[29] Pew Charitable Trust 2008: 15.   [30] Wuetrich 2003 and Smith, et al. 2009.

Economic arguments

One such argument is that intensive agricultural practices capitalize on economies of scale, and thus factory farming is a more efficient method of agricultural production than small-scale, local farming that minimizes animal suffering. Factory farming is the best way to produce protein-rich foods that most everyone can afford.

But is intensive agriculture really efficient? Some economists have said no, particularly when the full costs of industrialized animal production are brought into the equation – the cost of land use, particularly for waste disposal; the cost of air and water pollution; the cost to public health; and the cost to the community when property values and quality of life decrease. Corporate producers of animal products shift costs to neighbors and taxpayers, in general, and they also benefit from the existence of significant externalities, as well as government subsidies. They nonetheless claim that their methods of production are the most efficient. But the price of a pork chop or a chicken wing does not reflect the true cost.

A study undertaken in the United Kingdom by the Centre for the Environment and Society found the cost of cleaning up pollution, repairing habitats, and dealing with sickness caused by industrialized farming to be, "conservatively," 2.3 billion pounds, which almost equals the agricultural industry's income.[31] In the US, the cost of cleaning up air and water pollution created by CAFOs is usually paid by taxpayers in the county or state where the CAFO is located. When there is a clean-up, due to a spill or to the company having moved away, the costs are neither paid by the company responsible for them nor included in the price of the products they market. One of the ironies here is that vegetarians, who do not purchase industrially produced animal products, end up subsidizing those products if they pay taxes in a state or county where CAFOs exist. And citizens subsidize industrial animal production in many other ways, through direct subsidies from the government and through indirect subsidies such as rising health care costs.

Is vegetarianism ethically required?

The case against the industrial production of animals for food is strong on multiple grounds: humans, other animals, and our environments would

[31] Pearce 1999.

certainly benefit if factory farming ended. But what are we to think of eating animals that are not industrially produced? Do we have an ethical obligation to become vegetarians or vegans, regardless of how animals are raised and ultimately slaughtered? In most communities around the world people are in a position to make some choices about what they eat. As we have discussed in the last two chapters, in the absence of good reasons, one should refrain from harming those who can be harmed by ignoring their interests and denying them respect. Given that most humans do not need to consume animals, and culinary pleasures don't tend to be comparable to the values of life and liberty, we might think there is a prima facie reason for not raising and killing animals for food, whether they are raised in industrial agricultural conditions or not.

Of course, economic, legal, religious, and cultural forces construct and constrain our choices about what to eat, and choosing to forego consumption of other animals can be personally challenging as well. I've known many people who are vegetarian except when they go to their grandparents' house (to use just one example; it could be their aunt's house or their temple's Seder or their mentor's table and, of course, many vegetarians and vegans are grandparents!). Most people as guests in others' homes don't want to appear disrespectful, and one certainly doesn't want to get into a big hassle. For years, I dreaded going to my extended family's Thanksgiving dinner, because there would often be heated arguments about vegetarianism that were hard, especially since this was the only time each year that most of the relatives saw each other. Fortunately, there are now a lot of vegetarians in my family, and vegetarianism is no longer a source of uncomfortable discussions. Even when the conversations are difficult, or refusing to eat animals is awkward, most people, most of the time, can decide not to eat other animals, with relatively little effort. But there are cases in which there is more at stake than merely disrupting interpersonal harmony.

Contextual moral vegetarianism

Certain aspects of an individual's life, in particular contexts, may provide mitigating reasons against vegetarianism. Ecofeminists have long argued for a position called "contextual moral vegetarianism" that recognizes the ways that gender, class, race, ethnicity, and location can create genuine difficulties with choosing a vegetarian diet. Deane Curtin was the first to describe contextual moral vegetarianism when he realized that he could not "refer to an absolute moral rule that prohibits meat eating under all circumstances." If circumstances were such that he would have to kill an animal to feed his starving child, he readily admits that he would do it. And the acceptability of killing animals to eat them need not only exist in extreme cases of self-defense. There are people living in some parts of the world (for example, in arctic regions or deserts) and some engaging in certain types of cultural practices (nomadic traditions, for example) for whom a vegetarian diet does not make practical sense. It is not possible to cultivate plant food to sustain populations in the Arctic, and shipping tofu burgers to Inuit would ultimately harm more animals than those that are hunted and eaten. The "food miles" alone would contribute substantially to environmental destruction. It would also disrupt a sustainable way of life that allows humans and other animals, native to the region, to coexist.

Ecofeminists, and other theorists, have argued that context must play a role in determining whether or not other animals can justifiably be killed and eaten and are wary of the cultural imperialism that tends to accompany demands for universal ethical vegetarianism.[32] However, attention to certain climatic or cultural conditions does not amount to deference to all cultural practices. It is not a plea for moral relativism, where everything goes. Many traditions are oppressive not only to other animals, but often also to women and other humans who are thought of as different from those in positions of power and privilege, and who are also usually the ones identifying what practices constitute traditional cultural ones. Ecofeminists urge critical attention to the ways in which power may be operating to marginalize cultural "others," whether that means minorities, women, or other animals. They also eschew abolitionist approaches, like the animal rights approach, that require everyone in every context to become vegan, and argue that, in particular contexts, using other animals for food and clothing may be ethically justified.

"Humane" farming

The justification for taking the lives of animals to eat them will be strongest if the animals who are killed and eaten generally live their lives as they

---

[32] See, for example, Curtin 1991, Gaard 2002, and Gruen 2004.

choose and die painless deaths. This is often one of the articulated motivations behind what is sometimes called "free-range" farming or, more recently, "pasture-based" farming. As we've seen, the increase in industrial animal production has essentially wiped out small farms and ranches to the detriment of the animals and the environment. One former Montana rancher, who finds factory farming "unseemly and disquieting" in its reduction of animals to commercial goods, reminisces about his childhood on the family farm:

> On our farm with only a dozen or so of each [animal], many had names. They knew us and we them. (And people never ate anything that would come when called by its name.) We had expectations one for the other. When it was especially cold, my grandmother would warm the chickens' mash. Such behavior may seem silly, it surely was inefficient, but it seemed right then and I defend it now.[33]

There are some remaining small farms, and others have emerged, catering almost exclusively to their local communities, as people try to reconnect with their food and the land. These sorts of farmers focus on providing humanely cultivated, unadulterated food while building a sustainable connection to the land. They describe themselves as "beyond organic"; use no fertilizers, hormones, or antibiotics; and do not keep animals locked up. Tim and Liz Young describe their practices on Nature's Harmony Farm outside of Athens, Georgia this way:

> Our cattle forage on grass with sheep browsing what the cows don't eat. Chickens follow the grazers, spreading fertilizer naturally, and follow their instincts by foraging for insects and scratching on the ground. Our beautiful hardwoods are the perfect environment for rare breed pigs, who are free to use their terrific "plows" to hunt acorns, tubers and all kinds of great treats. Plus they help us by keeping everything clean and free of weeds.[34]

Like many in the new "locavore" and "slow food" movements, the Youngs see themselves as acting in harmony with nature and claim that "their animals are treated with love and respect and are free to naturally express their characteristics." The Youngs and others who have started pasture-based farms tend to follow the practices of one of the original grass-based operations, Polyface Farms, that prides itself on following "nature's template." For three

---

[33] Baden 1999.   [34] www.naturesharmonyfarm.com/natures-harmony-background/.

generations, the Salatin family of Polyface Farms has worked to "develop emotionally, economically, environmentally enhancing agricultural enterprises," and visitors, like writer Michael Pollan, claim you can't help but notice how happy the animals seem.[35]

Except, maybe, when the animals are about to be slaughtered. At Polyface Farms, chickens and turkeys are killed on the premises, and Joel Salatin is happy to let anyone watch. (Both Pollan and Salatin have argued for more transparency in the agricultural production process and wonder how that process would change if slaughterhouses had glass walls.) In the documentary film *Food Inc.*, there is a scene in which Salatin extols the virtue of killing animals in fresh air, with birds singing, and then commences the slaughter. If there are wild birds singing, they can't be heard over the screaming chickens that his crew grab, flip upside down, cram into killing cones, and then slit the throats of while the chickens are fully conscious. It is not an easy scene to watch. As one viewer noted, "When I watched this scene with an audience, I looked around to see that the vast majority of the crowd reacts viscerally: grimacing, covering eyes, wincing, looking away."[36] Watching animals being slaughtered is not usually a pleasing experience for the viewer, but it is undoubtedly much worse for those being slaughtered. *New York Times* columnist Nicholas Kristof, who often writes longingly about his boyhood memories growing up on a small family farm in Oregon, describes his experience as a child, killing geese:

> Once a month or so, we would slaughter the geese. When I was 10 years old, my job was to lock the geese in the barn and then rush and grab one. Then I would take it out and hold it by its wings on the chopping block while my Dad or someone else swung the ax. The 150 geese knew that something dreadful was happening and would cower in a far corner of the barn, and run away in terror as I approached. Then I would grab one and carry it away as it screeched and struggled in my arms. Very often, one goose would bravely step away from the panicked flock and walk tremulously toward me. It would be

[35] In *Omnivore's Dilemma* he writes: "To many animal people, even Polyface Farm is a 'death camp' – a way station for doomed creatures awaiting their date with the executioner. But to look at the lives of these animals is to see this holocaust analogy for the sentimental conceit it really is. In the same way we can probably recognize animal suffering when we see it, animal happiness is unmistakable too, and during my week on the farm I saw it in abundance." Pollan 2006: 319.

[36] http://civileats.com/2009/06/01/what-food-inc-can-teach-us-about-how-we-treat-animals.

the mate of the one I had caught, male or female, and it would step right up to me, protesting pitifully. It would be frightened out of its wits, but still determined to stand with and comfort its lover.[37]

On most pasture-based farms and other smaller operations, chickens, geese, turkeys, and other birds can be killed and processed on the premises, but, due to agricultural regulations, cows, pigs, sheep, and other animals are generally packed into trucks and shipped off to large slaughterhouses where, in the final hours of their lives, they are treated no differently than animals raised on factory farms.

Some pasture-based farmers take great pains to ensure that the animals they raise are killed with respect. Tim Young, for example, found a processor only an hour from Nature's Harmony Farm that kills only nine cows a day, compared to the 400 an hour killed in large processing plants. Slowing down the killing process minimizes fear and helps to ensure that pain is minimized. When possible, Tim is present as the cows are killed. As he puts it, he wants to "be there to look each one of my animals in the eyes so that they can at least have a familiar face." It is also his way of paying his last respects.[38] In order to avoid forcing animals to endure the terror of transport and slaughter at large plants, as well as to satisfy consumer demand for locally grown animal products, some farmers are hiring "mobile slaughterhouses" that come to the farm to kill and process the animals. One of these mobile units, owned by Lopez Community Land Trust, in Washington, is a specially equipped, refrigerated trailer that is pulled to the farm by a diesel truck. After killing the animals (only five to nine cows per day) the unit then drives the carcasses to a facility where they are cut into portions.[39] In California, another USDA-approved unit is operating. Elizabeth Poett of Rancho San Julian, an organic ranch with a cattle herd of 600, is proud to be able to use a mobile slaughtering unit, as it will provide the cattle with "more noble deaths and cut out the need for a long final slog in the back of a trailer to a far-off killing floor. It's a dream to be able to run this beef business like I've been able to do it with the mobile harvest unit. I sleep better at night."[40]

[37] Kristof 2008.

[38] www.naturesharmonyfarm.com/grass-fed-meat-farm-blog/2008/2/21/local-meat-processor.html.

[39] Etter 2008.   [40] Adelman 2009.

Replaceability

It appears that there are a number of farmers across the US who attempt to raise animals humanely, provide them with rich and satisfying experiences, allow them to roam with others of their kind, and then kill them painlessly. These are animals that would not have existed otherwise, and it could be said that their happiness adds value to the world. For those concerned about promoting happiness and minimizing pain – the hedonistic utilitarians we discussed in Chapter 1, for example – eating animals who are raised humanely and killed painlessly would not be ethically wrong.[41] For preference utilitarians, like Peter Singer, who judge actions based on the total amount of preferences satisfied over those thwarted, killing is objectionable only if that killing thwarts a preference or desire about the future, and, Singer argues, only persons can have preferences about the future. As we discussed in Chapter 2, persons have goals and projects that, for the most part, add meaning and value to their lives. A person may have a desire to write a book or make a film or adopt a dog or start an animal sanctuary in the future. The goals may be simple or grandiose, but, in either case, desires about the future would be frustrated if the person who had them was painlessly killed before she could act on those desires. Persons may also have desires for continued existence itself, and clearly that preference would be thwarted if a person were killed. In contrast, killing non-persons painlessly is not thought to be wrong, because non-persons do not have desires for, and preferences about, the future. Their lives can go better or worse, but their desires are immediate, about the here and now. They suffer from confinement and have desires to move around; they have desires for food and companionship; parents have the desire to nurture their offspring; and young have the desire to stay with their mothers. Denying animals freedom to move or to engage in species-typical behaviors and causing them physical pain are all objectionable for both classical and preference utilitarians. But there is nothing about killing non-persons that is ethically objectionable, as long as it is done painlessly. If the animal is standing in his stall, out of sight from others who might be

---

[41] Of course, it has to be true that the animals were raised humanely and killed painlessly for hedonists to accept the consumption of animals. Some have argued that it is not possible to do so and those that claim they are raising and killing animals humanely are perpetuating a myth in order to profit. See www.humanemyth.org/index.htm.

distressed to see him killed, and he is instantly stunned and then has his throat slit, nothing wrong has been done.

Yet, killing happy animals lowers the total happiness in the world. On both the classical utilitarian view and on Singer's view, painlessly killing happy animals should be ethically acceptable, other things being equal, only when those animals are replaced by equally happy animals. Indeed, as Singer writes:

> When we are not dealing with beings aware of themselves as distinct entities, the wrongness of painless killing derives from the loss of pleasure it involves. Where the life taken would not, on balance, have been pleasant, no direct wrong is done. Even when the animal killed would have lived pleasantly, it is at least arguable that no wrong is done if the animal killed will, as a result of the killing, be replaced by another animal living an equally pleasant life.[42]

Since farming is a business, in most instances, the animals killed are replaced by a new generation of animals that will also experience a happy life and then be painlessly killed. So, utilitarians would not object to eating other animals when they are raised and slaughtered humanely and replaced by more animals that will be raised and slaughtered humanely.

This replaceability thesis has raised a number of worries. One is that it leads to very counterintuitive results. Michael Lockwood discusses a scenario to illustrate the distasteful consequences of the replaceability thesis:

> Many families, especially ones with young children, find that dogs are an asset when they are still playful puppies (capable of keeping the children amused), but become an increasing liability as they grow into middle age, with an adult appetite but sans youthful allure. Moreover, there is always a problem of what to do with the animal when they go on holiday. It is often inconvenient or even impossible to take the dog with them, whereas friends tend to resent the imposition, and kennels are expensive and unreliable. Let us suppose that... people were to hit on the idea of having their pets painlessly put down at the start of each holiday (as some pet owners already do), acquiring new ones upon their return. Suppose, indeed, that a company grows up, 'Disposapup Ltd.,' which rears the animals, house-trains them, supplies them to any willing purchaser, takes them back, exterminates them and supplies replacements, on demand... Every puppy has, we may assume, an extremely happy, albeit brief, life – and indeed, would not have existed at

---

[42] Singer 1993: 132.

all but for the practice. Yet the activities of the company and its clients would, I imagine, cause a general outcry amongst animal lovers.[43]

And the counterintuitive results don't end with other animals. As we discussed in Chapter 2, there are many humans who are not considered persons as they do not have a sense of themselves as existing over time. They lack "self-consciousness," and thus, presumably, painlessly killing them and replacing them with other human non-persons who are at least as content as those killed would be acceptable. Of course, few would argue that this would be an acceptable source of protein, but given that there is a shortage of healthy organs for persons in need of them who often spend long periods of time in both physical and psychological pain waiting for a donor, the suggestion to kill human non-persons painlessly in order to provide organs to human persons is not patently absurd. And if we consider that there will be an increase in well-being and happiness for those who receive the healthy organs, then the need to replace the human non-persons (which raises all sorts of practical difficulties) would diminish. Utilitarians like Singer would argue that these sorts of ideas, if put into practice, would generate distress for many people and that distress needs to be taken into account in determining the permissibility of the action. Unlike the case of killing and replacing happy animals to eat them, which many people will find satisfying, killing and replacing happy human non-persons or puppies will not be met with the same reaction. There may be nothing directly wrong with killing and replacing human or canine infants, but there will be indirect harms and negative side effects that could outweigh whatever benefit is hoped to be gained.

But there is a more direct argument that might be made in response to the replaceability thesis. One might argue that even though happy chickens do not have explicit preferences for continued existence, they do, in fact, have future-directed interests. All admit that the animals that are typically raised and slaughtered to be eaten are conscious beings whose lives can go better or worse for them. They are intentional beings as well; that is, if permitted, they will move from one place to another on their own, will eat some things and not other things, will gather materials for nesting and pick a spot to build the nest, and will choose the company of some individuals and actively avoid others. Like human animals, other animals have identifiable desires and interests. And these desires and interests persist over time, although it is an

43 Lockwood 1979: 168.

empirical question just how long they do persist. When a cow starts to move to another part of the pasture, it might be said that she has an interest in getting to the spot where the grass is greener. If she is prevented from getting there, her interest or desire will be frustrated. If it is wrong, other things being equal, to thwart the future-directed desires and interests of persons, it is also wrong to thwart the future-directed interests of non-persons, although the wrongs may be of very different strengths.

The satisfaction of a chicken's interest in crossing the road or a cow's interest in moving to greener pastures requires continued existence. Those interests would not be satisfied if the chicken or cow were killed before getting to their destination. So, it could be argued, any diachronic interest is accompanied by an interest in living, even if the concepts of life and death are not ones that the individual possesses or is capable of formulating. Understood in this way, we can see what is wrong with the replaceability thesis. Because a puppy or an infant has an interest in being cuddled and cared for, she has a derivative interest in continuing to exist, and that interest is violated when she is painlessly killed. The same could be said for chickens, hens, sows, pigs, cows, and cattle. Their interests may not be as sophisticated as those of human persons, but they are beings that appear to have future-directed interests, even if their time horizon is rather short.

The category of edible

If we allow that raising happy animals and then painlessly killing them is wrong because it violates their interests, it seems that there is a philosophical argument for being a vegetarian beyond refraining from consuming animals raised on factory farms. Animal suffering matters and that is why one should avoid the products of industrial animal production. However, the other interests of animals matter too, and killing them to eat them, even if they are raised under ideal conditions, would violate those interests. But what if, as Jeff McMahan has recently asked, the animals are raised under conditions in which their well-being is promoted; they "die at a comparatively early age, when their meat would taste best"; and then we collect their bodies to eat once they are dead.[44] McMahan doesn't think it is "morally objectionable to eat an animal that has died of natural causes," and there are others who have

---

[44] McMahan 2008: 74.

advocated eating "road kill," animals who live in the wild but meet accidental deaths when they are killed by cars. Might there be an ethical objection
to consuming animals that are raised well or live free and die without our
intentionally killing them?

Cora Diamond, in a paper entitled "Eating Meat and Eating People," points
to a way we might think about what is wrong with eating animals that die
a natural (or accidental) death.[45] In her discussion of the ways in which the
typical arguments for animal "rights" go wrong, she claims the focus on
rights misses certain crucial facts about our relations to other humans and
to animals. She writes:

> We do not eat our dead, even when they have died in automobile accidents
> or been struck by lightning, and their flesh might be first class. We do not
> eat them ... We also do not eat our amputated limbs ... Anyone who, in
> discussing this issue, focuses on our reasons for not killing people or
> our reasons for not causing them suffering quite evidently runs a risk of
> leaving altogether out of his discussion those fundamental features of our
> relationship to other human beings which are involved in our not eating
> them. It is in fact part of the way this point is usually missed that arguments
> are given for not eating animals, for respecting their rights to life and not
> making them suffer, which imply that there is absolutely nothing ... at all
> odd, in the vegetarian eating the cow that has obligingly been struck by
> lightning. That is to say, there is nothing in the discussion which suggests
> that a cow is not something to eat; it is only that one must not help the
> process along.[46]

Humans are not food. Imagine how our interactions with one another might
be different if we saw humans, or at least some humans, as consumable.
If we saw each other as edible and, in fact, ate humans on occasion and
really enjoyed it, this could lead to a breakdown in respect for one another
and for humanity as a whole. Some feminists have argued that prostitution
has a similar impact on the value of women and on sexual activity. The
argument goes something like this: if sex from women can be bought and
sold, this diminishes the value of sexual activity and reduces women to sex
objects. Men who frequent female prostitutes have a tendency to treat sexual
activity as a recreational activity and are unable to see it as an intimate act.
Perhaps more importantly, these men tend to see all women, not just those

[45] Diamond 1978.   [46] Ibid.: 467–8.

who sell their sexual labor through prostitution, as less worthy of respect. Whether or not you think that prostitution is ethically objectionable, you can probably understand the logic underlying the argument. Once we engage in a certain kind of consumption, of women's sexual labor or of eating human flesh, when we allow certain things to be bought and sold on the market, we change the relationships we have and how we think of those relationships. We humans understand ourselves as not in the category of the edible, and this understanding, in part, shapes how we construct our relations with each other and the ways of life we share. If we now think of our bodies and other people's bodies as food, the value of our bodies and ourselves changes.

So, we might say that what is wrong with eating animals who live good lives and then die naturally (or accidentally) is that, in doing so, we don't respect them in the right way, as "fellow creatures," who, like us, do not belong in the category of the edible. Another way of putting this point is to say that in turning other animals from living subjects with lives of their own into commodities or consumable objects we have erased their subjectivity and reduced them to things. To do this is ethically problematic, because it miscategorizes them and perpetuates our own misperceptions. It also fore-closes another way of seeing animals, as beings with whom we can empathize and learn to understand and respond to differences. When we identify non-human animals as worthy of our moral attention because they are beings with whom we can empathize, they can no longer be seen merely as food.

That we can and do empathize with animals may have something to do with why so many of us may have difficulties with the idea of killing the animals we eat ourselves. As I said at the beginning of this chapter, there would probably be many more vegetarians if people had to kill the animals they eat. In some contexts, however, there are people who do have to kill the animals they eat, as it is often the only way they and their families can survive. In some of those contexts, the killing is done with empathy and reverence. Killing other animals for food does not necessarily mean that the animals are viewed as merely food, as just consumable objects. Many of those who hunt for subsistence have tremendous respect for the animals they kill, and the animals are honored as they are eaten. This suggests that it is possible to see other animals as individuals who are members of their own social groups, who have their own lives to lead, but who nonetheless can be killed out of necessity. In certain contexts, it is possible that humans will respect other animals as fellow creatures but also consume them.

There are not many contexts where it is necessary to kill animals for food in industrialized societies. However, as more and more people in cities are getting interested in the food they eat, many are rearing chickens and turkeys in their backyards. While some claim they are developing respectful, symbiotic relationships with animals before they kill them, it is important to reflect critically on the notion that these city dwellers are truly empathizing with the other animals and seeing them as fellow creatures. The rhetoric often used by urban locavores is that killing their own animals "teaches us humility and reminds us of our interdependence with other species." My suspicion is that the reaction to the killing is to become blasé. Slaughter is likely to require the killer to distance herself from the animal, much like the killers in the Tyson plants. One woman, reflecting on her first kill in her backyard (after admitting that she "kind of wanted to kill a chicken" and secretly hoping that the chick they named Arlene would turn out to be a rooster so she could kill him), described killing the rooster Arlene "as messy and mundane as cleaning the gutters."[47] Leaves and twigs and inanimate matter clog gutters; cleaning that away is a messy and mundane task, to be sure. Taking the life of a rooster, who was enjoying himself, pestering the hens, and making too much noise for the neighborhood, is different from cleaning gutters in so many ways. When they are experienced as the same sort of activity, with the same type of impacts, there is a failure of moral perception. In describing the killing of Arlene as akin to cleaning the gutters, the author not only saw Arlene as merely food and a nuisance to be cleared away, she seems to have missed the fact that he was a feeling being, with a life of his own, to whom moral attention was due.

Whether chickens and other animals are raised for food on factory farms, on pasture-based farms, or in urban backyards, and whether they live happy lives and die natural or accidental deaths, they are nonetheless individuals, with personalities and interests, relationships with others, and their own lives to lead. These are facts that warrant ethical attention. Without recognition of these facts and a significant reorientation toward other animals, ethical justifications for killing them for food, when it is not necessary to eat them, will remain questionable.

[47] Reese 2009.

4 Experimenting with animals

During the height of the Atlantic slave trade in the 1600s and 1700s, vervet monkeys, also known as green monkeys, ended up on ships sailing from Africa to the Caribbean Islands of St. Kitts, Nevis, and Barbados. The monkeys have since thrived on the islands. In fact, there are so many that most people view them as pests. Some people have found a use for the monkeys in biomedical research – in one series of experiments the monkeys have human stem cells injected into their brains to study Parkinson's disease.

In humans, Parkinson's disease is a non-fatal degenerative disorder of the central nervous system affecting an individual's motor skills, speech, and other functions due to loss of the neurotransmitter dopamine. The ability of a person to perform everyday activities and to participate as an active member of society generally diminishes as the disease progresses. In addition, the average life expectancy of a person afflicted with Parkinson's disease is commonly lower than for people who do not have the disease, because late-stage Parkinson's may cause complications such as choking, pneumonia, and falls that can lead to death. The number of people suffering from Parkinson's is increasing. A study of the five largest countries in Europe and the ten most populous countries in the world reports that there will be 8.7 million people with Parkinson's disease by the year 2030, a doubling in the number of those currently afflicted.[1]

In a laboratory on St. Kitts, researchers damage the vervet monkeys' brains, causing dopamine production to cease, in order to model human Parkinson's disease. Neural stem cells derived from human fetuses are then injected into the damaged monkeys' brains. After a period of months, the monkeys are killed, and their brains are removed and studied to see if the injected fetal stem cells have developed into dopamine-producing cells in the right part of

---

[1] Dorsey, et al. 2007.

the brain to compensate for damage.[2] Initial results were reported as "promising," suggesting that "the dopamine-depleted parkinsonian monkey brain" can "direct and sustain stem cell differentiation in ways that could be therapeutic for patients with Parkinson's disease."[3] In order for human stem cell therapy to move to clinical trials, specific new human cell lines would have to be created, so researchers have now developed human embryonic stem cells that they are testing on monkey brains with the hopes that, eventually, they will be able to implant human embryonic stem cells into human patients suffering from Parkinson's disease.

Inserting human embryonic neural stem cells into the brain of another primate creates what are called "chimeras" and this raises a number of ethical questions.[4] Technically, a "chimera" is an organism with two or more different populations of genetically distinct cells. Chimeras occur naturally, but most are created in laboratories. The term "chimera" originally referred to a menacing mythological creature, combining a snake, lion, and goat, and it may be this frightening association that leads some to worry about the sort of research that is happening on St. Kitts. Mixing human beings with animals evokes what bioethicists sometimes call the "yuck factor" – a reaction of unease or repulsion that signals that something is wrong even if we cannot yet quite say what it is. Some people worry that the monkey into whose brain human cells are injected will develop human cognitive capacities or in some other way become "humanized." The worst fear is that there might be a human person trapped in the body of a vervet monkey – that is, the vervet monkey would develop human consciousness – and this would raise serious ethical concerns about caging the monkeys, killing them, and ultimately removing their brains for study.

As we discussed in the first two chapters, ethical concerns about these invasive experiments should already have arisen, given that vervet monkeys are the kinds of beings who command our moral attention, even before the implantation of human brain cells. Vervets are socially complex, communicative animals who live in matriarchal family groups. They have distinct predator warning calls that alert others when a leopard, snake, or eagle is threatening. If a leopard warning call is issued by one of the monkeys, the

---

[2] Bjugstad, et al. 2005.   [3] Redmond 2008: 35.

[4] For a discussion of ethical issues about the use of embryos in stem cell research see Gruen, et al. 2007.

other monkeys head for the trees; if an eagle warning call is heard, they descend from the trees; and if a snake warning call is heard, they stand on their hind legs to search out the snake. Researchers observing vervets in their native African habitats have found that they are pretty clever monkeys. Marc Hauser recounts a fascinating incident:

> Tristan, the alpha male, pursued, groomed, and attempted to copulate with Borgia, the alpha female. After several tries … Tristan fumed and slapped Borgia on the head. Borgia screamed, causing all of her female relatives to come running. Within seconds, the Borgia family was chasing Tristan through the territory, weaving in and out of acacia trees. All of the sudden Tristan stopped, gave a loud leopard alarm call, and then sat and watched as the Borgia family fled up into the trees. Tristan remained on the ground … Tristan's alarm call appeared, on the surface at least, to be an elegant example of deception.[5]

Hauser never saw a leopard, but wondered why Tristan didn't complete the deception by climbing up the trees himself. We can't truly know whether Tristan made an honest mistake or figured out a clever way to escape a beating by the Borgia family. But other studies suggest that vervets and other social and communicative species are capable of manipulating others, a skill that requires relatively sophisticated cognition.[6] Vervets are sensitive primates with developed cognitive skills. They may be pesky to humans or each other, but they are creatures due moral consideration. Using them for research purposes raises ethical questions, whether or not the research is chimeric.

Conservative estimates suggest that globally at least 115.3 million animals are used in research, and an estimated 100,000–200,000 of these are primates.[7] Most of the experiments do not involve creating chimeras, although more research is being done in this area. At Stanford, for example, Irving Weisman is attempting to create a mouse with an entirely human brain. He believes that even if a mouse's brain consisted entirely of human cells it would still be a mouse brain in structure, form, and function. His hope is that the human cells that make up the brain would provide an excellent model for new treatments for human brain disorders. "If you have a human set of neurons – pain, hippocampus, learning, whatever – in the context of the mouse brain you could try a drug and say, What does this do to a simple learning task? What

---

[5] Hauser 2000: 156.   [6] Whiten and Byrne 1988.
[7] Taylor, et al. 2008 and Carlsson, et al. 2004.

does this do to perception of a smell – and so on." This would be a great improvement over using mice brains, as they are quite distinct from human brains, and the data gained from experiments on mice are not as reliable as they would be if the data came directly from human cells, tissue, and organs. Interestingly, Weisman himself admits that his hope of actually succeeding is dim. He thinks the most likely outcome of his research is that "it won't work at all. The most likely is that it won't repair the brain at all."[8] And this welcome honesty raises some of the central ethical questions for animal experimentation – if the data from animals is not as reliable as one would like and the experiments with animals are not likely to work, is using sensitive beings in perhaps painful, but always deadly, experimentation justified? Even if the information may be useful in promoting human and animal well-being, should we use other animals as a means to that noble end? Answering these questions is complicated, as there are a variety of different values at stake. Exploring the competing values and determining what research with other animals, if any, is justified is the goal of this chapter.

The pursuit of knowledge

Early experiments on animals were largely designed to obtain basic anatom-ical information. In a classic example of this pursuit, Galen, who lived in the Roman Empire in the second century, tied down squealing pigs, cut them open, and then severed their laryngeal nerves. Once the nerve was severed, the pig would continue to struggle, but the squealing ceased. At one of Galen's demonstrations in Rome, Alexander Damascenus, an "Aristotelian philoso-pher," heckled Galen claiming that we could not extrapolate from pigs to humans. He allegedly said, "Even if we are shown that sections of these nerves in animals render them mute, it is not necessary to believe it true in human beings."[9] At that time, it was widely believed that sensation, thinking, and talking all came from the heart. Galen's public, repeatable pig experiments established that, in fact, the brain controls behavior. In the sixteenth cen-tury, William Harvey did for the heart what Galen did for the brain. Harvey spent many years opening up and observing the inner working of snakes, rats, geese, snails, turtles, fish, deer, and dogs. His animal experiments revealed the

---

[8] www.pbs.org/newshour/bb/science/july-dec05/chimera_8–16.html.
[9] Gross 1998: 219.

nature of the circulatory system. Harvey established that, contrary to what was popularly thought, blood does not randomly float through the body, but is pumped by the heart through clear circuits of arteries and veins.

Though these early experiments involved cutting into living animals without any pain relief, as anesthesia had not yet been developed, important knowledge was gained. Nonetheless, the practice of "vivisection" was often viewed with great suspicion. Many objected to the cruelty involved. Others, like Damascenus, believed that there was nothing to be gained from studying animals as the results would have no application to humans. Still others worried about the arrogance, secrecy, and even sanity of those who engaged in the practice. Despite this skepticism, vivisection continued and eventually became standard practice in medical research. Claude Bernard's *Introduction to the Study of Experimental Medicine*, published in 1865, helped to establish animal experimentation as a central part of practicing science. Interestingly, while Bernard was heralding animal experimentation, his wife Marie-Françoise was one of his staunchest critics and objected to using animals on moral grounds. And she has company. Animal experimenters have critics in the sciences, as well as throughout society at large. Almost as soon as vivisection became common practice, anti-vivisection organizations emerged to try to end it.[10]

Beginning in the late 1800s, and continuing to the present, those who engage in animal experimentation and those who oppose it view each other with suspicion and derision. Vivisectionists were regularly characterized as ghouls, would-be Frankensteins, or unfeeling sadists. Critics of anti-vivisectionists characterized them as "soft muddle-headed women" and "sob-sisters."[11] Beyond the name-calling, there continues to be a serious struggle for popular approval and support by both sides. Those who oppose animal experimentation often characterize it in the press in the most disturbing of ways, and, as a result, those performing and defending the practice have developed techniques to obscure their research and deflect criticism.

In the early 1920s, the *Journal of Experimental Medicine* developed guidelines specifically to avoid criticisms from anti-vivisectionists. The journal required that specific language be used: "unanesthetized" rather than "no anesthetic"; "fasting" rather than "starving"; "hemorrhaging" rather than "bleeding";

---

[10] For an engaging discussion of the early history of reactions to vivisection see Rudacille 2000.

[11] Lederer 1992: 61–79.

"intoxicant" rather than "poison"; and "acute" rather than "severe." The journal wanted to avoid descriptions of suffering and encouraged the use of "impersonal medical terms." No details of animal distress or struggle during an experiment were to be described. Details of animal activity, distress, or vocalizations, before or during an experimental procedure, were to be eliminated. Susan Lederer, in her comprehensive study of the editorial policies at this journal, describes that in a 1935 article about experiments with cats, the editor instructed his assistant to change the text from "the brain was sliced off at various levels" to "the brain was removed." The journal would only print photographs when there was no way to describe them in words and, even then, would avoid printing photographs of the whole animal. They were particularly sensitive to any discussion of where animals came from (and, as we'll see below, they had good reason for that concern). They never allowed animals to be referred to by name and insisted on substituting the word "it" for "he" or "she." Lederer also found that the editor adopted strategies to try to make it appear that fewer animals were used. "For research reports involving dogs, monkeys, and cats the guidelines recommended that animal numbers be kept low and suggested renumeration or the substitution of letters and hyphens. For example, dog #897 would be referenced in the text as dog A8–97" to avoid the appearance that 897 dogs had been used.[12] A casual glance through the leading medical journals suggests that these obscurantist tactics continue today.

Many of the large research centers hire public relations people to deal with protests, as well as proactively to promote the results of experiments. I had a series of alarming encounters with a public relations employee at the Yerkes National Primate Research Center in Atlanta, Georgia. While doing historical, archival work on early chimpanzee research at the Manuscripts and Archives collections at Yale University and the Manuscript, Archive, and Rare Book Library at Emory University, I came across a number of photographs from the 1930s and 40s that I wanted to incorporate into my project.[13] When the Yerkes Center's public relations person found out about my work she closed the Emory archive to me and tried to get the Yale archivists to prohibit me from conducting further research. Ironically, in support of experimenters who want to be able to pursue knowledge without hindrance, this public relations person successfully hindered me from conducting my historical research.

[12] Ibid.: 74.   [13] See http://first100chimps.wesleyan.edu/.

The photographs that interested me were of chimpanzees who have long been dead. Nonetheless, the Yerkes Center was worried that this historical information would lead to protests, and I have been denied further access and information.

Changing attitudes and developing regulations

The medical research community has been very successful in maintaining a high degree of secrecy about their work and in preventing the public and our government representatives from getting involved in research regulation. This was less a problem in the United Kingdom, where they passed their Cruelty to Animals Act in 1876 and developed a more transparent system of animal experimentation. It took nearly a century before American legislation caught up in the form of the Laboratory Animal Welfare Act of 1966. The delay wasn't for lack of concern for animals in laboratories in the US. Antivivisection groups continually tried to bring the issue before Congress, but they were met by the powerful resistance of the "medical establishment."[14] That all began to change in the early 1960s as the popular press published stories about pets being taken from backyards and sent to research laboratories. One of the most gripping cases was that of Pepper, an adult, female Dalmatian who was taken from the Lakavage family's farm in Pennsylvania in the summer of 1965. The Lakavage family searched frantically for Pepper up and down the Lehigh Valley and even followed a lead to a dealer in upstate New York who allegedly obtained Pepper at an auction. After driving all day with her daughter and grandson in tow, Julia Lakavage was turned away at the dealer's property, but not before capturing the attention of Rep. Joseph Resnick. Representative Resnick, whose district contained the dealer's farm, was unable to help Julia and her family find Pepper, but he promised to take up their cause as "dog's best friend in Washington." It turned out that Pepper never made it to that farm. The dealer sold Pepper for research to Montefiore Hospital in the Bronx. While Julia and the family searched, Pepper was being cut open in an experimental surgery for pacemakers. She died on the operating table.

True to his word, a week after Pepper's death, Representative Resnick introduced a dognapping bill called "Pepper's Law" that garnered more public

---

[14] Stevens 1998.

attention than two historical pieces of legislation also making their way through Congress – the Voting Rights Act and Medicare.[15] In the aftermath of Pepper's demise, a group of activists that had been collecting stories of pet thefts for years was able to interest *Life* magazine in the growing problem of unscrupulous dealers stealing dogs and the unregulated facilities that were using those stolen pets in medical experiments. In February 1966, *Life* ran an eight-page essay with gruesome photographs entitled "Concentration Camps for Dogs" about one such dealer. A copy of the article was delivered to every member of Congress. Not long after, Pepper's Law was expanded from a proposal to prevent the theft of dogs and cats to a bill designed to regulate the treatment of all warm-blooded laboratory animals, whether stolen pets or not. That bill, the Laboratory Animal Welfare Act, signed into law in 1966, would later be known as the Animal Welfare Act (AWA).

The original AWA set minimum standards for the handling, sale, and transport of cats, dogs, non-human primates, rabbits, hamsters, and guinea pigs held by animal dealers. In order to prevent laboratories from experimenting on someone's companion animal, the law also required that dog and cat dealers who transported animals over state lines and laboratories that received federal money be licensed and provide identification records for the animals to ensure that they were not stolen. While this was a good start, as the public became more informed about the use of animals in laboratories, there was increased pressure to improve the 1966 AWA. The Act has been subsequently amended multiple times, in 1970, 1976, 1985, 1990, 2002, and 2007, and will, undoubtedly, be further refined.

The most significant improvements to the AWA came about in 1985 in the wake of a series of shocking revelations about conditions in laboratories brought to light by a new brand of animal activism. In the summer of 1981, a young college student named Alex Pacheco volunteered as a research assistant in a laboratory in Silver Spring, Maryland called the Institute of Behavioral Research. There, monkeys were surgically crippled so that they were unable to use certain limbs in an attempt to determine whether they could be rehabilitated. Pacheco documented the horrible, filthy conditions that seventeen monkeys were forced to endure and the painful procedures performed on them. He also took photographs. After a few months, Pacheco was convinced that the lab was operating in violation of a Maryland anti-cruelty statute,

---

[15] Engber 2009b.

and he brought his evidence to the police. The legal case against researcher Edward Taub on cruelty charges was the first of its kind, and although the charges against Taub were eventually dismissed (and, in 1990, the remaining monkeys killed), the case garnered tremendous media attention and subsequent public outrage. It also helped make Pacheco's newly formed animal rights organization, People for the Ethical Treatment of Animals (PETA), a serious force in the debate about the use of animals in research.[16] A few years later, in 1984, in California, at the Loma Linda University Medical Center, anti-vivisection protesters found unlikely allies – some members of the medical community, theologians, and both conservative and liberal journalists. All were condemning a xenotransplantation experiment in which a heart from a seven-month-old baboon was placed into a human baby. Baby Fae, as she became known, was born with a congenital heart defect, and doctors decided to try an experimental procedure, replacing her heart with that of the young baboon. Photos of Baby Fae, with a huge incision from her neck to her belly button, circulated around the world, and the experiment was met with disbelief by some, horror by others. Anti-vivisectionists, globally, called it ghoulish medical sensationalism. The medical community was divided, and many predicted that Baby Fae would die. Indeed, Baby Fae did die, when she was only three weeks old. In the wake of her death, there was added urgency for further regulation of medical experimentation.[17]

The 1985 amendment to the AWA, called the Improved Standards for Laboratory Animals Act, increased the power of the government to oversee animal research in laboratories and in other captive settings. It required the establishment of Institutional Animal Care and Use Committees (IACUCs) at all research facilities. These committees were to be made up of members of the research facility, attending veterinarians, and representatives of the public concerned for the animals' welfare, and their role was to review proposed research protocols to ensure that animal use was appropriate and that alternatives to the use of animals were explored. The amendment also required that dogs in laboratories get exercise and that researchers provide "a physical environment adequate to promote the psychological well-being of primates." It also specified that pain and distress be minimized in experimental procedures.

[16] Pacheco & Francione 1985.   [17] For more details see Mistichelli 1985.

Animal pain and psychological well-being

There was tremendous resistance by those involved in invasive animal experimentation to the 1985 amendment to the AWA. Once regulations were established that required exercise for dogs, environmental enrichment for primates, and minimization of pain and distress in experimentation, laboratory life would change significantly, probably more for experimenters than for those they experimented on. Many researchers, and even some philosophers, believed that animals are not capable of experiencing pain or distress, because animals do not have conscious experiences. To have a law on the books that actually requires that "psychological well-being" in primates be promoted and pain and distress be minimized meant that researchers had to give up their ideological commitment to denying animals have mental states. The law now establishes that animals' psychological states have to be taken into account. It may seem like common sense that animals feel pain, but, as Bernie Rollins notes, "Knowledge of and concern for animal pain was almost non-existent when the law passed."[18]

Pain involves both sensory and affective experiences. "Pain is not a reflex. It is a perceptual experience with powerful emotional and motivational components. Like all sensory systems, attributes of pain such as intensity, quality, duration, location, and extent depend upon cerebral processing."[19] The sensory experience, referred to as nociception, can occur without an affective or emotional component. An organism can feel a noxious stimulus but not experience pain. Some of those engaged in animal experimentation, and some of those who promote such experimentation, believe that animals are such organisms – they have sensory nerves that detect noxious stimuli but since they are not conscious they do not feel pain. Of course, experiences of pain are always subjective, and we can never exactly know what pain is like in another experiencing being. But, to deny that others feel pain because we can't directly experience what they are feeling is a mistake. There are two objective, or at least observable, ways to identify pain – one is physiological, the other behavioral. There is physiological evidence to suggest that all vertebrates, and perhaps some invertebrates, can experience pain because their nervous systems respond to noxious stimuli, and they have brain structures

18 Rollins 2006: 297.
19 Vierck, et al. 2008: 7–10. Their definition of pain "applies to both laboratory animals and humans."

that process nociception. Gary Varner has suggested that the presence of endogenous opioids, or pain-relieving endorphins, is another physiological indication that an organism experiences pain.[20] When the physiological evidence is combined with behavioral evidence, the case that animals feel pain is strong. The National Academy of Sciences identified a number of behavioral signs that can indicate an animal is in pain: guarding a particular area of the body, lack of grooming, altered facial expressions, altered behavior, disturbed sleeping patterns, altered social interactions, vocalizations, licking, biting, scratching, or rubbing the painful area, panting, sweating, and refusing food and water.[21] Knowing an animal's typical behavior helps one assess the degree of behavioral changes indicative of pain.

Of course, different individuals may behave differently to the experience of pain.[22] I know a chimpanzee named Juan who broke his leg so severely that a team of orthopedic surgeons had to implant a titanium rod to repair the spiral fracture. Before the surgery, Juan showed very little behavioral signs that he was in pain. Perhaps he knew that such signs would indicate to other chimpanzees in his group that he was weak and that may have led to further injury. Perhaps chimpanzees and other animals can intentionally mask their pain. In humans, we know that some individuals have a higher pain tolerance than others. Despite variability, the combination of physiological and behavioral indicators clearly supports the view that most animals can experience "conscious pain." As Fiery Cushman suggests, "There is little reason for us to doubt the existence of pain in many nonhuman animals besides the sort of brute epistemic skepticism that doubts if even fellow humans experience pain. Such skepticism has an appropriate place in philosophy, but strongly violates the principle of parsimony, which guides experimental science."[23]

Though a few people may remain skeptics about pain in other animals, there are many engaged in experimentation who are skeptical that animals experience psychological well-being. When the 1985 AWA amendment passed, most of those who performed experiments with primates balked. Of course, there are complexities associated with determining what counts as psychological well-being; as we've discussed, well-being can be understood subjectively, objectively, or by some combination, and figuring out what constitutes the well-being of other animals will require knowledge not simply about

---

[20] Varner 1998.   [21] National Research Council 2009: 50.
[22] Aydede 2006.   [23] Cushman 2006: 107.

species-typical behaviors, but also about individual personalities. Attending to a particular animal and understanding her behavior will help in an assessment of her interests and the promotion of her psychological well-being. This is a difficult and time-consuming method of assessment. And it is much easier to conflate physical well-being with psychological well-being, and some experimenters do just that, particularly those who want to justify the continuation of housing monkeys alone in cages. They suggest that when kept in isolation monkeys have a lower incidence of disease and wounds. Caged monkeys also show a lower incidence of joint disease than monkeys that are allowed to move around more freely.[24] However, some of the most ethically objectionable experiments with primates, involving psychological deprivation, showed that social primates suffer irreparable psychological damage when they are denied interactions with others of their kind.[25] The damage is particularly acute in infants reared in isolation. As one of the infamous experimenters who spent decades separating monkeys from their mothers noted, "By this ingenious research we learned what has been totally obvious to everyone else except psychologists for centuries."[26] The debates about the psychological well-being of primates bring to light a deep contradiction within animal experimentation – primates are similar enough to humans that experimenters use them as surrogates in psychological and other cognitive experiments, but when it comes to providing for their psychological well-being, experimenters deny that primates have psychological states. It is simply unscientific to deny that social animals suffer psychologically when they are not nurtured, when they are left alone and denied the opportunity to interact with others of their kind.

Despite the passage of the amended Animal Welfare Act, there are still thousands of animals that experience pain and distress in laboratories across the US, and there are hundreds of primates whose psychological well-being is not being promoted. Between December 2007 and September 2008, the Humane Society of the United States (HSUS) conducted an undercover investigation at the New Iberia Research Center, the largest chimpanzee research facility in the US, housing over 300 chimpanzees and 6,000 other primates.

---

[24] Kessler, et al. 1986: 769.

[25] See Davenport & Menzel 1963, Davenport, et al. 1966, Harlow & Harlow 1962, and Harlow 1974.

[26] Fedigan 1992: 210.

HSUS documented routine practices that caused physical and psychological distress, including chimpanzees in isolation cages measuring 5′ × 6′ for months at a time; monkeys and chimpanzees engaging in neurotic behaviors, including violent self-mutilation – ripping wounds open on their arms or legs; and infant monkeys separated from their mothers and isolated from them for weeks at a time. Since so much of what happens in laboratories is purposely kept from public view, investigations like that of HSUS or anecdotal reports are often the only way anyone not directly involved in animal experimentation knows what is happening behind laboratory doors. I was struck recently by an article entitled "Me and My Monkey: The Confessions of a Reluctant Vivisector," written by Daniel Engber, who before turning to journalism was a graduate student doing animal research. Engber's job was to bring Clayton, an adolescent rhesus monkey, from his cage to a restraining chair where his eye movements were recorded (through a device that was implanted into Clayton's skull). Engber quit graduate school "in 2003, after a grisly series of experiments involving a suction tube, a scalpel, and the exposed brains of a half-dozen Bengalese finches," but he stopped working with Clayton sometime in 2001. Eight years later, while preparing his article, he contacted his graduate school mentor to find out what had happened to Clayton. To his astonishment (and to mine as a reader), Clayton was still alive. Engber writes:

> In all the time I'd been gone, Clayton had lived in the same room, on the same feeding schedule, and with many of the same neighbors.... nothing has changed. Every day or two, he's carted off to a room painted all in black, and his head is fixed in place by the post that still protrudes from his skull... Clayton was born in a breeding center; he grew up in metal boxes and spent his adolescence with a hole in his head and a coil around his eye. In 10 or 15 years of life, he suffered through multiple surgeries and infections and endless hours of restraint in a plastic chair. And for what?[27]

It is hard to imagine that Clayton's psychological well-being has been much of a consideration to those legally bound to promote it. Though many had good intentions in working to pass the 1985 amendment, the Animal Welfare Act still represents minimal standards for animal welfare, does not even cover the vast majority of animals used in research, as mice, rats, birds, and reptiles are not considered animals under the Act, and the government has yet to question whether animal use in experimentation is ethically justifiable.

[27] Engber 2009a.

Weighing values

Since animal experimentation began, the public has asked whether the practice is justifiable. Some people, who do not believe that useful information
can be gained from experimenting on animals, answer the question with a
resounding "NO!" Yet, there is good evidence to suggest that we have learned,
and will continue to learn, from such experiments. While there are undoubtedly tens of thousands of animals who have suffered and died in laboratories
in useless experiments, it is also true that some animal experiments have led
to knowledge that has been central in the development of vaccines, pharmaceuticals, therapeutic procedures, and other protocols that directly improve
the well-being of humans and other animals. But is the fact that some benefits
have emerged from animal experiments enough to justify doing them?

When those who believe that experimenting on animals has led to some
benefits attempt to justify the use of animals, they tend to appeal, knowingly
or not, to a utilitarian or related consequentialist framework, one that tries
to weigh the beneficial consequences of experimentation with the costs associated with it. On this account, animal experiments are justified ethically
when the well-being of humans, and perhaps other animals, is enhanced
by experiments that were done with the fewest number of animals possible
experiencing the least amount of pain and suffering. Given that human disease causes so much suffering, if that suffering can be minimized by causing
less suffering in medical experiments, then a utilitarian would probably find
those experiments justified.

A controversy about the adequacy of the utilitarian approach to animal
experimentation erupted not long ago in Britain's popular press. At issue
was a supportive comment utilitarian philosopher Peter Singer made in a
British documentary about the research of Tipu Aziz, a scientist who performs primate neurological experimentation at Oxford University.[28] Aziz,
like the researchers on St. Kitts, creates brain damage in monkeys in order
to mimic the symptoms of Parkinson's disease. In his experiments, Aziz confines monkeys in primate-restraining chairs, drills into their skulls, implants
electrodes, performs other electrical and surgical manipulations, and then
observes their behavior for a period of time before killing them to remove
and study their brains. According to the *Guardian*, Aziz claims that 40,000

[28] *Animal Testing – Monkeys, Rats and Me.* 2006.

people around the globe have benefited from the techniques he has developed, and only 100 monkeys have been sacrificed.[29] For a utilitarian like Singer, if there were no other way to obtain this benefit, including the possibility of experimenting with fewer humans at a similar cognitive level to monkeys, then he would agree that it was a justifiable experiment.

I call Singer's test for when an experiment on a non-human animal is justified the "non-speciesist utilitarian test" or NSUT. According to NSUT, an experiment X would be justified if and only if:

1. Of all the options open, X generates more pleasure or benefit than pain or cost on balance; and
2. The justification for experiment X does not depend on irrelevant species prejudice, that is, equal interests are considered equally no matter who has them.

This framework has often been lauded for its simplicity and its practical usefulness. It apparently allows one to make a relatively clear determination about whether an experiment might be justified. In order to reach a conclusion about any particular experiment, one has to measure and compare pleasures and pains across species to know that this was the only way to achieve a balance of pleasure over pain and to establish that the use of animals was not based on speciesist reasoning.

There are familiar objections to part 1 of NSUT, which is a straightforward utilitarian position, and there have long been utilitarian responses to the objections. There are also problems that emerge in the interpretation of part 2. Let's consider two familiar objections to part 1 – the incommensurability objection[30] and the epistemic objection or the cluelessness objection[31] – in the context of stem cell research, in order to see the kinds of problems one particular case can raise for NSUT. Then we can turn to examining worries about part 2.

Since initially formulated, consequentialist theories that rely on being able to make interpersonal utility comparisons – that is, to compare the well-being of one person with the well-being of another and make judgments about the weight of a good for some versus the weight of a harm for others – have been

---

[29] Jeffries 2006.

[30] Although often referred to in this way, the issue here seems to be, as Ruth Chang suggests, really one of incomparability. See Chang 1997.

[31] Lenman 2000.

scrutinized.[32] It is often claimed that values are incommensurate, and thus meaningful comparisons cannot be made. It is hard enough to compare our own pleasure playing pushpin to our delight reading poetry; the exuberance of watching the Colts win the Super Bowl with the passion in seeing Venus Williams win at Wimbledon. How then are we supposed to compare the benefits a human gets from reading about Victorian gender relations with the benefits a dog gets catching a Frisbee? Since utilitarian theory relies on making just these sorts of comparisons, critics contend that utilitarian theories cannot guide our action.

In response, consequentialists have pointed out that, whether or not we are any good at it, we make these kinds of comparisons all the time in our daily lives. John Harsanyi suggests that the basic intellectual operation in making such comparisons is "imaginative empathy." When we are deciding between actions that will affect two different people we try to put ourselves into both those individuals' positions, with their sets of interests and desires, to figure out the effect the action in question will have by their lights. Once we have done that, we can determine which course of action will lead to the most benefit (or, perhaps, least harm) and take that action. The more we develop our empathetic skills, and the more we learn about those around us who we are likely to affect more of the time, and about people generally, the better we will be at making these interpersonal utility comparisons.

This seems to be true when deciding which of one's children should get the bigger piece of pie, or which friend should get the theater tickets you are unable to use. But what about those cases in which the ethical stakes are quite high and the deliberation impersonal, as is often the case when thinking about such issues as animal experimentation? Consider one type of stem cell research designed to reverse the damage from spinal cord injuries (SCIs). The goal is to develop stem cell therapies that could eventually be used to replace destroyed nerves, to create supportive tissue environments

---

[32] Harsanyi sugests that "the long-standing opposition by many philosophers and social scientists to interpersonal utility comparisons goes back to the early days of logical positivism, when the role of nonempirical *a priori* principles, like the similarity postulate [the assumption that, once proper allowances have been made for the empirically given difference in taste, education, etc., between me and another person, then it is reasonable for me to assume that our basic psychological reactions to any given alternative will be otherwise much the same (639)], in a choice among alternative empirical hypotheses was very poorly understood." Harsanyi 1977: 641–2.

to allow for axon regeneration, and to replace the myelin-forming cells that allow signaling along surviving axons. Such therapies, in principle, could help some reasonably large percentage of the roughly 8,000 people in the US, alone, who have suffered spinal cord injuries. Approximately 55 percent of these injuries are classified as incomplete injuries, signifying that these individuals experience varying degrees of constant pain in addition to the loss of mobility and function.[33] Most people are unaware of the fact that so many people with spinal cord injuries, even those who are paralyzed "from the neck down," experience pain, often excruciating neuropathic pain that most of us have never felt. Accurate empathy, in this case, requires fairly extensive study of spinal cord injuries and getting to know people who have experienced them. People involved in rehabilitation and care for those living with SCIs are in the best position to engage in this sort of imaginative empathy and can inform the rest of us. Those people doing research, particularly basic research on stem cells, often are not directly in contact with those suffering from spinal cord injuries, so their claims as to the extent of the potential benefits will generally not be as accurate as those who have more extensive knowledge of the particular suffering SCI survivors experience. Because SCIs vary so widely, determining the full nature and severity of the harms the injuries have caused to each individual and their families, friends, and support networks is also a challenge. Yet, despite the difficulties of trying to get a handle on the shape and intensity of the suffering in order to make interpersonal utility comparisons, it is not hard to conclude that eliminating or minimizing the suffering caused by SCIs would be a very good thing to do.

But, in order to do that very good thing, a vast amount of pain and suffering has to be inflicted deliberately on animals, the majority of which are rodents. (However, dogs, cats, and primates are also used in SCI research.) Animals used as models in SCI research generally have weights dropped onto their spines to cause precise types of injuries in particular locations. There is no way to obtain a reasonable estimate of the number of animals involved,[34]

---

[33] According to the 2000 SCI database the most frequent neurological category at discharge is incomplete quadriplegia (34.1 percent), followed by complete paraplegia (23.0 percent), complete quadriplegia (18.3 percent), and incomplete paraplegia (18.5 percent).

[34] One could, presumably, go through every article that was ever published on the topic and count the number of animals reportedly used in the protocols and then go to the articles referenced and count the number of animals used there, and the number used in the references cited, etc. This would provide some data, yet there are hundreds of experiments

but a conservative estimate, useful for illustrative purposes, would be that, at the very least, 80,000 animals annually will have to be experimented on and killed in the development of stem cell therapies for SCI. Animals have been, and will continue to be, used in the development of SCI models; in developing and refining various transplantation protocols; in generating neural stem cell progenitors and other cell types for transplantation; and in the stem cell transplantation protocols themselves. Training, modifications in procedures, and duplication of results will also involve the use of animals. And, of course, this does not include the animals that were used in the early basic research that led to increased understanding of both spinal cord function and mammalian developmental processes, as well as of the pluripotency of embryonic and fetal stem cells in the first place. If we suppose that, in ten years time, this use of animals will lead to a stem cell therapy for those humans suffering SCIs; that the human therapies will improve once human clinical trials and treatments are in place; and (quite unrealistically) that animal experiments for SCI treatments at that time will stop, we can – again, for illustrative purposes – say that, if this research is successful, the use of approximately 800,000 animals will lead to improvement in quality of life for people suffering spinal cord injuries into the future.

Can we compare the suffering and death of the animals used in the development of stem cell therapies for spinal cord injuries with the suffering of those individuals who suffer from SCIs and that of their families and friends? If we assume that 8,000 individuals suffer and survive SCIs per year and that the animal suffering is equivalent to human suffering, it would take 100 years to benefit 800,000 SCI sufferers. But, clearly, that isn't the right equation. The animals used may suffer horribly in the experiments, but their suffering comes to an end when they are killed. The benefit accrued to humans, whose suffering will presumably end with the successful development of stem cell therapies, is the avoidance of an average of twenty or so more years of pain and suffering. And there are other factors that make such comparisons troublesome. Humans suffering from SCIs don't just experience pain, but also depression, frustration, anger, grief, humiliation, and other taxing emotions as a result of being incapacitated, to varying degrees, by their injuries. They are

in which animals are used that never get written up for publications. Because rodents, birds, and reptiles are not covered under the AWA in the US, there are no data about their use, which further complicates making an estimate.

also dependent on others who will suffer emotionally, and those dependent upon individuals who suffer SCIs will also suffer. Importantly, individuals who suffer SCIs can currently treat most of their pain and many, if not most, people suffering SCIs can achieve significant forms of independence allowing them to lead meaningful lives. Animals in spinal cord research generally do not have their pain relieved adequately, and there is no goal, such as independent living, for them to reach toward, and no pleasure in their short lives.

Comparing the benefits to humans who have suffered spinal cord injuries to the harms of those animals used in research, as part 1 of NSUT would have us do, is not straightforward, even when making specific (though unrealistic) assumptions about success and about numbers, as I have done here. Spinal cord injuries are complex, and, as one specialist recently acknowledged:

> [while] stem cell transplantation in mice and rats with partial spinal cord injuries has demonstrated improvement in locomotor functions, investigators have recognized that they must overcome biochemical inhibitors, provide appropriate growth factors at the correct time, while directing structural growth. The human central nervous system – the brain and the spinal cord – is 10 times the length of a rodent's. To allow for healing you must cover ten times the distance that is present in rats and mice. Making the jump from the animal model to the human model is a fairly large leap.[35]

And herein lies another problem with part 1 of NSUT for practical deliberation – how do we know when we are justified in saying that, of all the options open, conducting these spinal cord injury experiments with animals will lead to the development of stem cell therapies that will benefit individuals with SCIs?

This "epistemic objection" has long plagued utilitarians – how can one know, in advance, what the consequences of one's actions will actually be? In most animal experimentation the goal is to gain information about basic biological processes, not to lead to any particular therapeutic consequence that will immediately or obviously change the world for the better. The suffering that is caused to animals may not even be expected to lead to any benefits down the road; as experimenters like to say, scientific research is not linear. Often unexpected knowledge is gained from experiments. Part 1 of NSUT

[35] American Academy of Physical Medicine and Rehabilitation 2006.

suggests that, because we can't know what benefits might result from basic research, but we do know about the negative consequences in terms of animal suffering and deaths that are directly caused by the research, we would never be justified in supporting any basic research and that even comparative judgments between different types of basic research cannot be made. Consider a decision to use twenty sheep in a basic research experiment designed to get some ideas about whether there is a part of the brain that contributes to homosexual behavior, or to use sixty mice to try to figure out the mechanisms of diabetes. In neither case is there a clear or immediate therapeutic goal; experimenters are just trying to learn more about biological processes. NSUT would thus say neither is justified. However, it does seem that in the case of the homosexual sheep experiment, the question itself doesn't warrant either the use of scarce financial resources or the use of animals, whereas the case of diabetes might. Even in the context of basic research with animals, we can make distinctions between projects, but NSUT doesn't provide us with guidance in making those distinctions, because no benefits are being promised.

Since it is not just hard, but in many cases impossible, to answer the question, "is performing experiment X the only action that will lead to greater benefit than the harms it causes?" it appears that part 1 of NSUT does not provide the kind of practical guidance in particular cases that we would expect from a theory that is meant to be practical and action-guiding. This difficulty becomes accentuated when we turn to the second part of the test. Even in those rare cases when we have an affirmative answer to part 1, in order to consider an experiment ethically justified, part 2 of NSUT must also be satisfied. Engaging in non-speciesist reasoning to determine the right animal model for a particular experiment involves considering the use of human animals as well as non-human animals. There is great scientific value to using humans as bio-models for human disease and injury, as the problem of extrapolating from one species to another would be avoided. Currently, clinical trials serve this function, as they are experiments on humans that occur after particular treatments have been tested on non-human animals but before the drug or therapy is released for use to the general public. Part 2 of NSUT suggests that human animals be considered earlier in the experimentation process.

Part 2 of NSUT would have us determine whether the decision to use mice, dogs, cats, and non-human primates was made without species prejudice.

One way to accomplish this is to consider equal interests equally and, as Singer has suggested, we can do this by asking "whether the experimenter would be prepared to carry out the experiment on human beings at a similar mental level." Another way to do this has been proposed by Ray Frey. He has us consider the quality of life of the individual in question, whether human or non-human. He writes, "Not all lives are of the same value...if we have to take life, we should take lives of lesser value, other things being equal...I know of nothing that cedes any and all human life greater value than any and all animal life."[36]

To understand fully what this would mean, let's return to the stem cell research example for spinal cord injuries and again assume, for the sake of argument, that current research will lead to therapies in a decade or so that will allow people who suffer SCIs to recover both function, including mobility, and normal sensation. This would mean injuring the spinal cords of human experimental subjects who are at a similar "mental level" or "quality of life" to the non-human subjects, thus creating extraordinary pain in cases of purposely generated incomplete injuries. Pain relief will be withheld some of the time as it would interfere with the experimental protocol, and, for some of the induced SCIs, adequate pain-relieving pharmaceuticals have yet to be developed. It will also involve the introduction of neural progenitor embryonic stem cells into the spinal column. Initially, these cells may grow in inappropriate places or form tumors, leading to additional spinal cord damage and additional unrelievable pain. At some point, these human subjects would be killed and their spinal cords studied, as would be the case with the non-human animal subjects. As per our assumption above, after a decade or so, the technique would succeed and stem cell therapies would become available to people suffering from SCIs from that point forward. People, who would otherwise spend their lives confined to wheelchairs and in pain, would be able to walk, and their pain would be minimized if not eliminated. If we assume that fewer human experimental subjects would be needed than non-human subjects – let's say only 8,000 over the ten-year period, or 800 a year, which would be one hundred times less than the number of non-human animals proposed – would we be prepared to engage in the research?

This proposal should give us pause. As we discussed in Chapter 2, when analyzing the Argument from Marginal Cases, there are two ways to evaluate

---

[36] Frey 2002: 46.

this sort of proposal. One is to accept, as Frey does, that experiments on animals and on humans are ethically justified. The other is to recognize that, insofar as we are unprepared to use human beings in spinal cord or any other painful experimentation, we should reject the idea that the research can ethically be performed on animals. As Singer has said, if a researcher using non-human animals is not prepared to use, for example, humans born with irreversible brain damage, then they are engaged in speciesist reasoning, and their experiments would not pass part 2 of NSUT.

So while, in the abstract, many would endorse the utilitarian justificatory scheme when it comes to animal experimentation, it looks as though the theory does not justify, and perhaps cannot justify, most of the current uses of animals in medical experiments.

Abolition of animal experimentation

There are some people who object, in principle, to the utilitarian approach that would allow the possibility, however remote, that experimenting on animals is ethically justifiable. Like the utilitarians, the abolitionists hold that animals have lives that can go better or worse for them, that they should not suffer unnecessarily, and that they deserve to have their interests taken into consideration. Unlike utilitarians, however, abolitionists never think it is appropriate to use another individual as a means to one's own ends. Even if it is clear that the experiment would end more suffering than it would cause, it still would not be justifiable. There are three interrelated arguments that support the abolitionist position.

When we use others as means, we reduce them to instruments, and their value is based on how they serve in that role. Opponents of using animals in experimentation reject the notion that animals can or should serve as "model organisms" for human disease. Animals have their own lives to live and distinct ways of living those lives, all of which is denied them when they are seen as tools for research. Some have argued that the best way to see what is wrong with a view that reduces sensitive beings or subjects-of-a-life to tools or instruments is to consider cases in which individual humans were so reduced. The Nazi hypothermia experiments are often raised in this context. During the Second World War, Nazi soldiers faced hostile thermal environments, and there was very little information available about what the human body could withstand. Soldiers were being shot down over the North Sea, and the military needed information about how long they might survive in the cold water and how to warm them if they were rescued. Similar problems were faced by soldiers in damaged U-boats. In order successfully to rescue and ensure the well-being of the troops, the German government endorsed hypothermia experiments on human prisoners in Dachau.[37] The experiments happened because "science rationally devalued [certain] human beings to the point where their only value was as physiological or anatomical specimens."[38] Even if they led to useful medical knowledge, the Nazi experiments were widely condemned as an affront to humanity. Nazis failed to appropriately value the lives of human beings. Those opposed to animal experimentation argue that the intrinsic value of animal lives is not being recognized in an analogous way. It's a mistake of ethical perception, a type of "blindness," that undermines our moral agency and our own animality.

However, under certain circumstances, we do allow experiments on human beings, and, when we do, we don't necessarily devalue the human subjects. This is because the only experiments with human subjects that are ethically acceptable are those done with the subject's full and informed consent. This wasn't always so. Between 1932 and 1972, in Tuskegee, Alabama, poor African Americans with "bad blood", actually syphilis, were used in experiments to track the progression of the disease for the US Public Health Service. Early in the study, in the 1940s, penicillin became the standard treatment for syphilis, but experimenters not only failed to provide penicillin and information about its curative affect to the men in the study, but they also prevented them from getting treatment anywhere. A quarter of the men in the study died of syphilis; many of their wives contracted the disease; and some of their children were born with congenital syphilis, which is life-threatening for infants. The subjects in the study were not informed about the nature of the study, and, in fact, they were being harmed by it. In the 1960s, another egregious set of experiments was performed, this time with a group of mentally retarded children living at the Willowbrook State Hospital in New York. The children were deliberately infected with hepatitis A and then treated in various ways. The facility would not admit new patients unless the parents consented to the experiments.[39]

When these studies came to light, Congressional hearings were held, and, ultimately, laws were established to provide protection for human subjects,

---

[37] Pozos 2003.   [38] Ibid.: 455.   [39] Murphy 2004.

emphasizing the importance of respecting persons by requiring informed consent, minimizing risks to subjects, avoiding coercion and conflicts of interest, and requiring heightened scrutiny for any research on vulnerable populations. Those seeking to end experimentation with animals argue that because an animal can never give consent and because they have been historically oppressed and undervalued, they are a particularly vulnerable population and thus should not be used for research purposes, and that there should be strict regulations in place to protect them.

It is interesting, in thinking about the argument for informed consent, to consider that laws protecting human embryos from use in experimentation in the US currently are far more stringent than any regulations governing the use of animals. Animals cannot give verbal consent, nor can embryos. But we might think that existing animals would object, if they could, to being used in experiments. They would object to being held in cages, often in isolation; being subjected to invasive procedures; being denied the opportunity to exercise the capacities that are constitutive of their well-being. It makes little sense to think that embryos in Petri dishes, qua embryos, could similarly object, yet they have greater legal protection. Part of that protection is due to human exceptionalism that elevates the value of human life, even *in vitro*, over the value of other animals' lives; part comes from the institutional desire for people, in this case embryo donors, to have full knowledge of what sort of research they are consenting to. In the US, using federal funds for experimentation that involves creating embryos for research is prohibited. Federal money can only be used for research on human embryonic stem cell lines that were created from "excess" embryos created for reproductive purposes as long as the embryo donors provide full and informed consent to have the embryo destroyed in order to be used for research. There are few, if any, restrictions on funding for animal research.

The third type of argument that those seeking to abolish animal experimentation make is based on a view about the limits and stringency of ethical demands. There is a general moral presumption by those who do not hold utilitarian views that one should never be morally required to suffer for another, particularly if that suffering involves extreme sacrifice. Even utilitarians tend to limit ethical sacrifice to things of "comparable moral worth." Although it may be laudable for an individual to give up all her worldly goods for the sake of animal protection or to feed the hungry, it is not ethically required. It is a commendable choice one may make, but it is supererogatory, it goes beyond what any reasonable ethical theory can require. Since the animals who are used in experimentation do not benefit from it, indeed they are usually killed, this sort of sacrifice runs counter to the presumption against incurring the suffering of one individual to benefit another. Insofar as we think it is wrong to require someone to give up an organ for another in need, or to require transferring all of one's disposable income to provide education for every child, abolitionists believe it is wrong to force animals to endure experiments that will not directly benefit them.

When we take these three arguments together and when we look at the practical difficulties with the utilitarian position, it does indeed seem that the moral weight is heaviest on the side of ending research with animals. This has already happened with chimpanzee experiments that are now outlawed in every country in the world, except the US. In 1986, the British government banned the use of chimpanzees in research on ethical grounds, arguing that given how close chimpanzees are to humans, to treat them as expendable is immoral. The last research facility using chimpanzees in Europe stopped in 2004, when biomedical research with chimpanzees became illegal in the Netherlands. Japan ended biomedical experimentation on chimpanzees in 2006. Apparently, many countries have recognized that some research is beyond what a decent society can endorse. When we consider the vast and expensive infrastructure of animal experimentation, the vested interests of those engaged in animal use becomes rather clear. Virtually every scientific article ends by claiming "that more research is needed." This is how research scientists make their livings. There is little motivation for seeking alternatives, much as in the energy industry that has relied so heavily on fossil fuels. As long as animal interests are not taken into account and experimenters are unmotivated to change, it seems ethically reasonable to oppose animal experimentation.

5   Dilemmas of captivity

In 1953, in the forests of Sumatra, Indonesia, a five-year-old elephant, later named Shirley, was captured and sold to the Kelly–Miller Circus. As of this writing – fifty-seven years later – she is still alive. During her first twenty-five years in captivity, she was a circus performer. In 1975, while performing for the Lewis Brothers Circus, Shirley was attacked by another elephant, and her right back leg was severely broken and never properly healed. After performing for two more years, even with her badly injured leg, she was sold to the Louisiana Purchase Gardens and Zoo in Monroe, Louisiana where she remained for over two decades, chained by the hind leg, without other elephants. Shirley did have a compassionate human caregiver, Solomon James, who looked after her at the zoo for the next twenty-two years.

Then, in 1999, it became clear that Shirley would do better living with other elephants and with space to roam, so the zoo retired Shirley to the Elephant Sanctuary in Hohenwald, Tennessee. There she would be able to spend the rest of her years roaming over hundreds of acres with other female Asian elephants. She was accompanied on her trip from Louisiana to Tennessee by her caregiver, Mr. James, and the event was videotaped for what would become an Emmy-award-winning documentary by Allison Argo entitled *Urban Elephants*. The scenes of James saying his farewell are unforgettable. As he gave Shirley her last hose bath, with tears in his eyes, he removed her ankle chain. He said, "Shirley girl, I don't know who the first person was that put this chain on you, but I'm happy to be the last to take it off. You are free at last." He kissed her trunk, told her he was going to miss her, and left her to begin the rest of her life.

Elephants are highly intelligent, social animals who form close family ties. In the wild, their social structure is matriarchal, and they live in small groups of between six to eight adults with an experienced female leading the family unit. Groups usually consist of the daughters of the matriarch and their offspring, but non-related females and their young may also be part of a family unit. Female elephants maintain lifelong bonds with their family group, and they remember each other, even when separated for years.

Not long after Shirley and James parted, the power of elephant memory was on full display. As a young calf, decades earlier, one of the Asian elephants at the sanctuary, Jenny, had been with Shirley at the same circus. According to the sanctuary co-founder, Carol Buckley:

> Jenny came into the barn and . . . There was an immediate urgency in Jenny's behavior. She wanted to get close to Shirley who was divided by two stalls. Once Shirley was allowed into the adjacent stall the interaction between her and Jenny became quite intense. Jenny wanted to get into the stall with Shirley desperately. She became agitated, banging on the gate and trying to climb through and over.
>
> After several minutes of touching . . . through the bars, Shirley started to ROAR and I mean ROAR – Jenny joined in immediately. The interaction was dramatic, to say the least, with both elephants trying to climb in with each other and frantically touching each other through the bars . . . We opened the gate and let them in together . . . they were as one, bonded physically together. When one would move, and the other would move in unison . . . All day they moved side by side . . . This relationship is intense and resembles that of mother and daughter.

Shirley and Jenny, though separated for twenty years, were now insepara-ble at the sanctuary, even through Jenny's very last days. Jenny, though much younger than Shirley, came to the sanctuary in 1996 in very ill health. Jenny recovered enough to fully enjoy each day of her remaining ten years at the sanctuary, but the physical toll of her early life was inescapable. During the last week of Jenny's life, in October of 2006, Shirley was at her side, helping her to get up when she could. When it was clear that Jenny's life was coming to an end, Shirley walked off into the woods and stayed there. She didn't eat for two days. Fortunately, Shirley had bonded with other elephants, and they helped her heal.

In the wild, elephants spend most of their day walking, often covering vast distances. By contrast, elephants in captive settings are rarely provided enough space to roam. Elephants used in circuses (and some zoos) are almost constantly chained by both a front and a back leg to prevent escape. These heavy chains often damage the elephants' legs, preventing the elephants from getting the daily exercise they need. Coupled with uncomfortably hard floor-ing, these conditions cause many captive elephants to develop debilitating arthritic conditions and other painful foot and leg ailments.

Circus elephants and some elephants in zoos are trained by techniques that involve aversive or painful stimuli, including electric shock, whipping, and physical force. The "bullhook" or "ankus" is one of the more extreme devices for getting elephants to submit to the will of a trainer. Trainers embed the hook in the soft tissue behind or inside the ears, inside the mouth, and in tender areas around the feet. The hooks are intended to cause sharp and intense pain and act as a behavioral stimulus so that the massive animals will comply with the trainers' commands even after the hooks are removed. Often, just before a performance (and out of sight of circus goers), trainers will inflict a few painful "reminders" to ensure that the elephants perform on command.

Controversy over keeping elephants in captivity has grown in recent years as more is learned about these highly intelligent, sensitive individuals who can live sixty or more years. Scientists observing elephants in the wild have been documenting the effects that poaching has on the members of a family who witness a slaughter. They have observed a measurable increase in unpre-dictable social behavior, depression, hyper-aggression, and levels of stress hormones in some of the elephants studied. This has lead scientists to posit that elephants, like humans, can suffer from post-traumatic stress disorder or PTSD.[1] Because elephants are so social and require years of socialization in their maternal family units, develop lifelong bonds, and have strong mem-ories, disruptions in their social group, such as that caused when family members are killed or when youngsters are captured for captive purposes, have deep psychological and behavioral effects. Being held for decades in cir-cus or zoo environments, away from family members, with few opportunities to develop social relations with others of their kind, traumatizes elephants.

Though the Association of Zoos and Aquariums (AZA) has begun to set standards for elephant care that recommends larger herds be maintained, that female elephants should not be alone, and that more complex and larger enclosures be provided, these are just recommendations, and many accredited facilities do not meet them. There are no guidelines for providing for the psychological well-being of elephants in circuses. So elephants remain in

---

[1] Bradshaw, et al. 2005: 807.

inadequate captive settings and are forced to suffer for decades. Some zoo keepers are recommending publicity campaigns to try to convince the public that more elephants should be captured in the wild and brought to zoos. Two prominent zoo advocates recently wrote, "due to the high profile elephants now have with animal rights activists, there may be increasing legal and political barriers to elephant importation. This makes it especially important that zoos become more proactive in . . . building the case for elephants in zoos."[2] Despite these attempts, elephant experts and animal advocates will continue to argue that keeping large, long-lived, socially complex, highly intelligent animals such as elephants in captivity is wrong.[3]

Elephants are just one of hundreds of types of animals that are our captives. As we discussed in the last two chapters, billions of animals are bred, reared, and ultimately slaughtered for food and millions are kept and killed for scientific experimentation. Animals are also kept in a wide variety of captive settings for different purposes. Some animals are held captive to fight with humans in bullfights or each other in dog or cock fights. Some are captive performers – they are made available to star in television shows, commercials, or movies; to appear at town festivals or at birthday parties; they are hauled from city to city to perform in circus acts or other spectacles; or they wait in tanks or cages until it is time to perform in-house. Some animals are held captive at roadside attractions. Others are on display in zoological parks and aquariums, some of which are accredited, some of which are not. Some animals are kept captive to race or to hunt. Some are kept captive and then are ultimately skinned to provide human clothing. Various types of animals are kept in our homes as companions, as guards, as curiosities. Others live in sanctuaries or refuges.

To hold someone captive is to deny her a variety of goods and to frustrate her interests in a variety of ways. Though conditions of captivity vary considerably, I think it is most useful to think of captivity as a condition in which a being is confined and controlled and is reliant on those in control to satisfy her basic needs.[4] Animals respond differently to being captives.

---

[2] Hutchins and Keele 2006: 219.

[3] For a range of views see Wemmer & Christen 2008.

[4] It would be more precise, but bulky, to specify that "normally functioning adult beings" are considered captives when they are confined and controlled and reliant on those in control to satisfy their basic needs. People who are incarcerated in prisons are captives; dependent children and those human adults with severe cognitive disabilities are not generally

Domesticated animals like dogs and cats who live as our companions can have rich, happy lives in captivity if they are well fed, have companionship, exercise, and otherwise have their interests satisfied. As we have seen, other domestic animals raised and slaughtered for food and those used in laboratories have miserable lives, full of suffering, and we can only imagine that death is a relief for them. Wild animals have varying degrees of difficulty existing in captivity. Elephants, marine mammals, and many birds simply cannot thrive as captives. Others suffer from species-specific forms of stress, injuries, human-contracted disease, and boredom. As a recent study notes:

> In the wild, an animal can generally move away from aversive light or sound; it can seek shelter from undesirable climatic conditions, dig into the earth to cool itself, and time its daily activities to coincide with whatever environmental variables are most suitable. The captive animal, however, has no such luxury. In general, animals in captivity have little or no control over the timing, duration, and/or nature of the light, sound, odors, or temperatures to which they are exposed. For the most part, this lack of control is a direct result of confinement.[5]

Given that most conditions of captivity cause inescapable physical or psychological suffering, we might think that unless there is a very good reason for holding animals captive we should release them. However, in the case of many, perhaps most, captive animals, release would be a death sentence. As we'll see in the next chapter, many of the wild counterparts of animals living in captivity exist precariously because their habitats are being destroyed at alarming rates. In many cases, there may be no wild left into which the captive animals can be released. More importantly, even if there are environments into which captive animals may be returned, most captives have lost the ability to survive on their own in their native habitats.

The story of Keiko, the orca whale who starred in the movie *Free Willy*, is one cautionary tale. Keiko was born in the Atlantic Ocean and captured when he was just two years old. He was held in an aquarium in Iceland, sold to an aquarium in Canada, and then sold to an amusement park in Mexico

thought of as captives, as they are unable to care for themselves. Even though they might be denied the same freedoms, in the case of children and severely cognitively impaired individuals, it is for their own good. Some assume that keeping normally functioning adult animals in captivity is for their own good, but this is a more contentious claim.

[5] Morgan & Tromborg 2007: 277.

City. While in Mexico, he starred in the movie and became somewhat of an international celebrity. Like the story in the movie, children and marine mammal advocates campaigned to free Keiko. A foundation was formed and work began to rehabilitate Keiko at a facility in Oregon with the hope of eventually releasing him to the ocean. When he was twenty years old, he caught his first live fish after extensive efforts to teach him to hunt for his own food. Eventually, Keiko was returned to a large bay off the coast of Iceland, not too far from where he is believed to have been born. Marine mammal specialists continued to try to teach him the ways of wild orcas, and, gradually, over a four-year period, he was reintroduced to free-ocean living. The worry was always whether he would be able to feed himself and handle himself with other orcas. He did have contact with others of his kind and swam the oceans free of human contact for about two months, but his life as a free whale was short-lived. He soon followed a fishing boat into a Norweigan fjord where he again sought care from humans. Though he was free to leave, he chose to stay, and shortly thereafter died at about the age of twenty-five, apparently from pneumonia.

The difficulties of reintroduction to the wild are many, and success rates are low.[6] Most current captives are the products of many generations of captive breeding, and it is unclear that humans would be able successfully to rehabilitate and introduce these captives to free living. In addition, many captive social animals form deep bonds with those with whom they share an enclosure, when they are lucky enough to have companions. Ripping them away from their captive companions and moving them to new environments may not be in their best interests.

The fact that so many animals are currently living in captivity poses an ethical dilemma. Keeping animals captive, confined, and controlled, and denying them freedom is, other things being equal, generally thought to be wrong. In this chapter, we'll explore the philosophical arguments that suggest how and why captivity is wrong. If it is wrong, then, on one horn of the dilemma, we find that we may be doing something wrong by visiting zoos, having pets, and

---

[6] The average rate of success ranges, but apparently never goes above 50 percent. Differing definitions of success also make generalizing about reintroductions difficult. In the case of Keiko, for example, reintroduction of an orca had never occurred before and for some involved in the effort, that he was able to live in the ocean and make choices about where to go constituted success, even if he ultimately chose the company of humans and did not survive long. See Fischer & Lindenmayer 2000.

supporting sanctuaries. But, releasing animals from captivity will make them worse off and may even lead to their deaths. This other horn of the dilemma is ethically problematic too. At the end of this chapter, we will assess whether or not there is a reasonable way to resolve this dilemma, but, before we do that, we will want to examine three quite different captive contexts – zoos, homes, and sanctuaries – and the particular ethical challenges each raises. Do we cause animals to suffer needlessly by keeping them captive? Do we violate their liberty? Do we undermine their dignity? Answering these questions will help us determine whether it is possible to escape the ethical dilemma that animal captivity poses.

Zoos

Wild animals have always been kept in menageries of some form or another, but it wasn't until the mid-eighteenth century that the precursors of the modern zoological parks that display captive animals for public amusement and education emerged. The first such zoo is thought to be Tiergarten Schönbrunn, or Zoo Vienna, which opened in 1752. The London Zoo opened almost a century later in 1847 and served as a model for many of the zoos in Europe and in the US. There is some dispute about which was the first zoo in the US – the Philadelphia Zoo or the Lincoln Park Zoo in Chicago. The Philadelphia Zoo was chartered in 1859 and opened to the public in 1874 with a relatively large collection of animals. The zoo boasts that in its first year of operation it had 813 animals and received well over 228,000 visitors. They charged a quarter for adult admission and a dime for children. The Lincoln Park Zoo considers itself the "oldest free public zoo" in the US and notes the donation of a pair of swans in 1868 to mark its inception. In 1874, the Lincoln Park Zoo bought its first animal, a bear cub, for $10. Around this time, interest in zoological parks was growing, and it was not long before zoos opened in many major cities across the US. By the turn of the twentieth century, there were zoos in New York City, Buffalo, Cincinnati, Binghamton, Baltimore, Providence, Cleveland, Portland, Atlanta, St. Louis, Milwaukee, Denver, St. Paul, Omaha, Pittsburgh, Washington, DC, and San Francisco.[7]

Most of the animals that lived in these early zoos were kept in cramped cages, enclosures, or tanks, often alone, indoors or with limited access to fresh

[7] Robinson 2004 and Hanson 2002.

air and sunlight, and these captives did not live long. If they survived for longer periods, they developed abnormal behaviors, referred to as stereotypies, such as pacing, hair-plucking, head-rolling, and rocking. Essentially, very little was known about how to care for wild animals. As David Hancocks notes:

> [Z]oo managers and designers . . . knew virtually nothing about the wild habitats of the animals or of their natural diets, their breeding habits, natural groupings or lifestyles. Bread and milk mixed with boiled rice was the staple diet for numerous species in most zoos. The daily ration for the elephant at the *Jardin des Plantes* was eighty pounds of bread, twelve pints of wine, and two bucketful of gruel.[8]

In the early days of zoos, though visitors were amazed and amused by what they saw, they often complained about terrible smells, flies and filth in cages, and lethargic animals.

As zoos became more established, some zoo directors began experimenting with enclosure design and the ways that animals were displayed. In Hamburg, in 1907, Carl Hagenbeck opened two innovative "panoramas," an "African" panorama and an "Arctic" panorama, in which animals from each geographical area were displayed in a created environment with geological features modeled on those found in native landscapes.[9] Another important innovation was to remove the bars separating the animals from the zoo visitors and installing moats instead in an attempt to make the experience more naturalistic. Zoos around the world started to copy these ideas, although there were some who argued strongly for continuing to organize zoos taxonomically – for example, by having a primate house, a snake house, an aviary, etc. – and who believed that providing greater space with natural features would allow the animals to hide from zoo visitors. The zoos that did try to replicate the open panorama model often did this without the forethought put into the original in Hamburg. "At its worst, and sadly most common, this resulted in mere heaps of stones cemented together with little similarity remaining to the original structures."[10] Enclosure improvements continued in fits and starts as more was learned about caring for animals in captive settings and

---

[8] Hancocks 2003: 55.

[9] Of course, Africa is a huge continent with very different environments. In more recent times, the geographical exhibits are more specific. For example, you might see the African savanna or the African rainforest.

[10] Hancocks 2003: 67.

as public attitudes were changing. In the 1960s, some zoos started to arrange animal exhibits according to animal behavior to serve an educational role by, for example, creating birds of prey areas and dark houses for nocturnal animals. By the turn of the twentieth century, as environmental destruction and animal welfare became more pressing public concerns, some zoos created "immersion exhibits," described by the St. Louis Zoo as "a lushly planted naturalistic environment that gives visitors the sense they're actually in the animals' habitats. Buildings and barriers are hidden. By recreating as many sights and sounds as possible from natural environments, immersion exhibits provide an exciting experience and educate visitors about how animals live in the wild."[11]

Changes in how zoos display animals often resulted from shifting justifications for the existence of zoos. Initially, zoos were designed to amuse, amaze, and entertain visitors. Exhibits made the animals accessible to the gaze of the zoo visitor, and there was little context for understanding what was being seen. As attitudes about animals and their environments started to change, even better zoos could no longer be justified solely on recreational grounds. Few zoo directors today would appeal to the recreational value of a zoo experience to justify the expensive maintenance of zoos, particularly when there are so many other ways for families to spend an entertaining day together. Nonetheless, recreation continues to play some part in justifying zoos. The AZA describes zoos as "popular family fun" and boasts that, in 2008, 218 AZA-accredited zoos and aquariums attracted more than 175 million visitors, approximately 50 million of whom were children, "making accredited zoos and aquariums some of the best places for families to connect with nature and each other."[12]

Research, conservation, and education have replaced entertainment as more central justifications for zoos. Yet, research done in zoos raises an obvious question about precisely what is being studied. Behavioral research, which is the primary type of research undertaken at zoos, is problematic, as the behaviors of captive animals are quite different than the behaviors of their wild counterparts; so what is being learned, if anything, is what an animal does in captivity. This sort of knowledge has certainly helped zoos maintain animals in better conditions, for longer periods of time; but, as Dale Jamieson

---

[11] www.stlzoo.org/yourvisit/thingstoseeanddo/riversedge/immersion.htm.
[12] www.aza.org/about-aza/.

puts it, the "fact that zoo research contributes to improving conditions in zoos is not a reason for having them. If there were no zoos, there would be no need to improve them."[13]

Zoo conservation efforts don't provide the best justification for keeping animals captive either. Although there are a few zoos that have done important work funding research and conservation efforts in habitat countries, most haven't. Of course, there are many organizations that support conservation efforts that do not also hold animals captive. Over the past twenty years, there has been a great deal of discussion about the role that zoos play in saving endangered species, but few animals have been saved from extinction by zoos, and "some of them more by providence than prudence."[14]

The zoo community has recently argued that their goal is not primarily direct conservation, but rather they see themselves as a major force in educating zoo visitors to become actively engaged in conservation efforts. As a 2007 AZA report stated, "Zoos and aquariums all over this country are making a difference for wildlife and wild places by sharing their passion for conservation ... By creating interactive exhibits, interpretive tours and educational programs that bring people face-to-face with living animals, zoos and aquariums profoundly influence their visitors in significant ways."[15] The report was based on a three-year study that was the first to attempt to measure the effect that visiting a zoo had on attitudes toward conservation. While widely heralded as an important project, the methodology of the study has come under scrutiny. Critics report that there is "no compelling or even particularly suggestive evidence for the claim that zoos and aquariums promote attitude change, education, and interest in conservation in visitors ... Only well-controlled research, not enthusiastic assertions ... can address the question of whether claims concerning the positive effects of zoos and aquariums on visitors are justified."[16] More research may help, but a look to what zoos are doing to "improve" provides a different picture.

The Dallas Zoo has recently spent $30 million to construct "Giants of the Savanna" a multi-acre enclosure in which giraffes, elephants, ostriches, zebras, and other animals will mix in a naturalistic landscape that simulates their native habitat. One might expect this highly touted innovation to contribute to the conservation education mission of the zoo, to encourage zoo

---

[13] Jamieson 2002: 170.   [14] Hancocks 2003: xviii.
[15] Falk, et al. 2007: 5.   [16] Marino, et al. 2010: 126–38.

visitors actively to engage in conservation efforts. But, in fact, it will encourage visitors actively to engage with the captive animals as entertainment. The animals will be trained to perform "naturalistic" behaviors during peak visiting times. "Animal activities will be strategically scheduled throughout the day, keeping the animals active and drawing people through the habitat." It will not be completely naturalistic, however, as people will be able to buy biscuits to feed the giraffes. Zoo director Gregg Edwards claims, "It's not a passive, 'let them out and loaf' kind of exhibit. It's a kind of habitat theater."[17] With these sorts of innovations one wonders if zoos are teaching the right thing. Jamieson has argued:

> Zoos teach us a false sense of our place in the natural order. The means of confinement mark a difference between humans and animals. They are there at our pleasure, to be used for our purposes. Morality and perhaps our very survival require that we learn to live as one species among many rather than as one species over many. To do this, we must forget what we learn at zoos. Because what zoos teach us is false and dangerous, both humans and animals will be better off when they are abolished.[18]

There are currently more than 800,000 animals in AZA-accredited facilities. That is a large number of captives. Even if evidence does emerge that zoos can teach the right things and have a positive impact on attitudes about conservation, they would also have to show that holding so many animals captive is the only way to impact conservation efforts in order, ultimately, to justify their continued existence.

Zoos are not going away any time soon. Even if the practice of breeding to sustain captive populations was abandoned, many long-lived animals will be in captivity for quite some time. For some species, like chimpanzees, remaining in zoos may be a good thing, or at least the best option given the situation, as there really is nowhere else for them to go; for elephants, continued captivity isn't as good, as there are no zoo environments adequate to satisfying their need for space and companionship. Let's suppose, in contrast to reality, that there was enough knowledge, money, and will to create captive environments in which all captives had their needs met – high-quality food they enjoy, protection from predators, good company, enough space to engage in a variety of species-typical behaviors, the ability to avoid stressful stimuli, and

[17] Fluck 2010.   [18] Jamieson 2002: 175.

provisions that prevented separation from their group or their being sent to other facilities for breeding purposes – would keeping animals in captivity be acceptable? In other words, if we imagine that captive animals won't suffer physically or psychologically, is there anything wrong with captivity itself?

Liberty

We might think that even though the animals are being treated well and aren't obviously suffering psychologically or physically that there is still something wrong with keeping them in captivity. In our hypothetical idealized situation, we are imagining that the animals do have their needs satisfied and they aren't suffering, yet their liberty is being denied. Being denied liberty, other things being equal, is generally thought to be ethically problematic. But what makes denying individuals their liberty wrong? In order to answer this question, we need, first, to be clear about what having liberty means and why it is valuable.

Liberty can be understood in a variety of ways – sometimes it is thought of as the state of being free from restraint; sometimes it is thought to be our ability to control our actions; and sometimes it is thought of as an absence of arbitrary interference. John Stuart Mill in *On Liberty* says, "Liberty consists in doing what one desires," or, presumably, being free to do what one desires. We often think of liberty as the freedom to make choices and often those choices are between competing desires. When we are free, we not only make choices, but also voluntarily act on those choices. Even when we decide not to do something, we act on that choice by voluntarily refraining from doing it. When our options are constrained or when we are coerced to do one thing, like it or not, then our liberty is being violated. Of course, our options are always constrained by what is possible; we are not free to do anything imaginable. I am not free to hold my breath and swim across the English Channel underwater as a fish might, or to fly across the channel on my own as a gull might. That I do not have those options doesn't mean my liberty is being infringed upon.

Denying liberty or depriving someone of her freedom, which is what captivity does, is thought to be one of the things that can make a life go badly for that individual. There are two ways that denying individuals their liberty can negatively impact their lives. If we understand liberty to be an instrumental value, then respecting an individual's liberty is important because it is *conducive* to other things that are valuable, like pleasure and well-being. Doing what one wants, being free to make choices and to act on them, following the desires one wants to satisfy, and not being interfered with in the pursuit of one's desires, are all freedoms that are important, because they contribute to making an individual's life go better by allowing that individual to satisfy her desires. Individuals who are confined, restrained, or subordinated cannot act freely upon their desires and live their lives as they want. Liberty can also be thought of as an intrinsic value, a value that in itself, regardless of anything else, makes a life valuable. Liberty in this sense is *constitutive* of living a good life. Let's look at both of these ways of understanding the value of liberty to see how captivity may undermine each.

Allowing individuals to choose what they want and not interfering as they pursue that choice leads to the satisfaction of an individual's own desires, and that is, generally, thought to be good for them. Individuals are in the best position to know what they want, and allowing individuals the freedom to try to satisfy their desires is valuable. It is true that having the liberty to follow one's desires may not always, in fact, be conducive to flourishing. As we discussed in Chapter 1, sometimes an individual might have desires that, if satisfied, do not actually enhance well-being at all. I may really want to eat a whole chocolate cake. It may be the strongest desire I have, and I am free to eat it. If I do, however, I may not feel so well afterwards, and my desire to eat it and the freedom to act on that desire might end up not promoting my well-being. My late dog Buddy would eat whatever stinky thing he found, and when he was free to do so (because I couldn't or didn't stop him) he would then throw up and mope around with a stomachache. When he was free to act on his immediate desires, his well-being wasn't actually promoted.[19]

Conversely, well-being might be experienced in the absence of liberty. I may think that my well-being is being promoted because I have altered my desires to fit my unfree conditions. For example, someone may have distorted preferences that are shaped in response to her oppressive or confined situation. The subordinate "happy" housewife who accepts abuse and blames herself when her domineering husband is angry that the house isn't cleaned exactly the way he likes is one example. Some Marxists and feminists call this "false consciousness," a state in which a person comes not only to accept

---

[19] In acting on these immediate desires I am assuming that these are not uncontrollable urges. My eating the chocolate cake and Buddy's eating whatever he finds are not, for the sake of this argument, the actions of a wanton. See Frankfurt 1971.

her unfree condition, but also believes that her life is going well. Economists call these "adaptive preferences" and suggest that under certain types of oppressive or liberty-denying social arrangements, the people being denied liberty adapt their preferences to suit their lack of freedom. Similarly, living a free life may contain all sorts of hardships, and being kept safe, well fed, and protected from danger may promote well-being, even while freedom is denied. So liberty may not always lead to flourishing.

If liberty is just a useful tool for promoting interests, then it seems that if there is some other way to promote those interests, then liberty isn't particularly important. This strikes some theorists as mistaken. The value of liberty, they argue, goes beyond its role in allowing us to satisfy our desires and to fulfill our interests. Leading a genuinely good life involves the actual satisfaction of interests we both want satisfied and that turn out to promote our flourishing. The process of satisfying our own interests is valuable in itself. If this is right, then we must be free to make the right choices about what is good for us, by our own lights, and actually pursue those choices free from interference and, with luck, satisfy them. We must be the ones who control the process that leads to our well-being. Liberty can be conducive to well-being (but isn't always) but liberty is always constitutive of a genuinely good life, one in which an individual's actions are under her control.

It is important here to note that in trying to establish that liberty is intrinsically valuable we should not diminish the importance of other aspects of well-being that are necessary for living a good life, such as being free from pain and distress and having adequate food and shelter. If an individual's liberty is denied, that does not necessarily mean that life is a bad life or a life not worth living, as that individual may have other intrinsically valuable components of her life in place. If I was to imagine myself in the science fiction world we discussed in Chapter 1, where I have been taken away by aliens, and we think of the captors as benevolent beings who provide me with most everything I want – say, good food, comfort, companionship, health care, entertainment, intellectual stimulation, etc. – my life can be thought to be a good one, certainly worth living. These things are all constitutive of a good life for me. It would be a better life if I were actually able to provide myself with these things and was free from captive control, however loving or kind it may be.

As we discussed, keeping animals in actual captive conditions often causes them to suffer injuries and other physical harms. The stress, stereotypies, and other psychological harms that captives experience often are the direct result of their instrumental liberty interests being violated. They are not free to choose when to eat or who to spend time with or where to nest; they cannot avoid noise or light; and burrowing animals often can find no comfort. All of these deprivations cause them to suffer. It is at least conceivable, if not ever fully practical, that, like the benevolent aliens, we humans might be able to provide an idealized captive environment for animals. Since they care about being free from physical and emotional pain; they want good food, comfort, health care, entertainment, and stimulation; and social animals want and need companionship; if we were to provide all these things, giving them the freedom to avoid stress and satisfy their interests, would denying them their liberty by keeping them in captivity still be wrong? In order to answer this question, we need to determine whether other animals have an interest in liberty as such, an interest that is violated when they are held captive. In other words, are any other animals the sorts of beings who can be said to value liberty intrinsically?

Autonomy

Some would argue that in order to have an interest in liberty as such, to recognize liberty as intrinsically valuable, that individual would have to be the sort of being who not only values freedom from physical and psychological pain and the satisfaction of her desires, but also is capable of a type of second-order valuing. This sort of individual recognizes herself as an agent who is free to make choices and to act on those choices or not, and values that capacity as an expression of herself. Some philosophers have suggested that this capacity is part of what it means to be autonomous. Another way of putting this is that to be autonomous an individual must create her own conception of what would constitute a good life for her, be able to revise that conception as new information and new desires emerge, and be able to pursue that conception. Alasdair Cochrane has argued that most captive animals are not autonomous in this way and do not have an intrinsic interest in liberty, thus pain-free captivity is not objectionable. He writes:

> Most animals cannot frame, revise and pursue their own conceptions of the good. This is not to say that sentient animals do not have different characters, nor is it to deny that they can make choices. It is simply to make the point that most animals cannot forge their own life plans and goals. Given this, restricting the freedom of these animals does not seem to cause harm in the

same way that it does for humans . . . As autonomous agents, most human beings have a fundamental interest in being free to pursue their *own* life plans, forge their *own* conception of a good life and not to have a particular way of life forced upon them. However, in the case of a horse used in show jumping, the restriction of freedom seems less obviously harmful. Since they lack autonomy, horses are not able to forge and pursue their *own* conceptions of the good. In which case, it is unclear why restricting the freedom of the horse and imposing a way of life on the animal is necessarily harmful. This, of course, is not to say that interfering with horses or preventing them from having control over their lives *never* causes harm. Obviously, if we were to train the horse using violence, if we failed to keep the horse in a suitable environment or if we were to make the horse perform dangerous tasks, then harm would be done. However, the harm in such cases is caused by the suffering to the horse, not the lack of liberty itself. For this reason, it seems initially plausible to propose that for non-autonomous animals, their interest in liberty is only instrumental, whereas for autonomous humans it is intrinsic.[20]

Conceptions of the good life

Is Cochrane right that animals lack an intrinsic interest in liberty? Are no other animals autonomous individuals who have a conception of the good life and the ability to act on that conception? In order to have a conception of any-thing, one has to have concepts. Comparative psychologists, philosophers, and cognitive ethologists have tried to determine whether or not non-linguistic beings have concepts. Some argue that without language one cannot have thoughts and thus cannot have concepts. Donald Davidson argues in this way. He suggests that other animals do not have concepts, because in order to have a concept one must have a certain kind of knowledge – namely, knowledge of how one concept relates to other concepts and beliefs. He writes:

> To have the concept of a cat, you must have the concept of an animal, or at least of a continuing physical object, the concept of an object that moves in certain ways, something that can move freely in its environment, something that has sensations. There is no fixed list of things you have to know about, or associate with, being a cat; but unless you have a lot of beliefs about what a cat is, you don't have the concept of a cat.[21]

[20] Cochrane 2009: 669.   [21] Davidson 1999: 8.

But if animals lack concepts, then what is one to make of the various experiments that have been performed in which animals are able to match words to images or objects? For example, in experiments with pigeons, the birds were shown a variety of photographs and were trained to peck at the pictures that had trees, but not to peck at the pictures in which there weren't trees. Once they correctly mastered the task and understood what photographs to peck at, they were given new photographs, some that contained trees and some that didn't, and they only pecked at the photographs in which there were trees. This might suggest that they understand the concept of "tree."[22] You'll recall Sarah, the chimpanzee discussed in Chapter 1, who not only matched symbols to objects and understood the difference in meaning when the symbol order changed, but also seemed to understand that pictures represented objects, and not just any objects, but those required to solve a particular problem. She was shown videotapes of a human actor trying to solve a problem and then was presented with two photographs, one of which represented the solution. If she did not have a concept of both the problem in need of solution and how the photograph represented the solution, how was she able to make the correct selection with such high frequency?

Some might say that this ability to match solutions with pictures or to discriminate some pictures from others doesn't require concept possession. Humans can put various things in the right categories without understanding the concepts behind the discrimination. As Davidson puts it, "A creature does not have the concept of a cat merely because it can discriminate cats from other things in its environment. For all I know, mice are very good at telling cats apart from trees, lions, and snakes. But being able to discriminate cats is not the same as having the concept of a cat."[23]

Colin Allen has a different way of thinking about concept attribution. He says we would be right in attributing a concept X to an animal, human or non-human, when:

i. The animal systematically discriminates some Xs from some non-Xs; and
ii. The animal is capable of detecting some of its own discrimination errors between Xs and non-Xs; and
iii. The animal is capable of learning better to discriminate Xs from non-Xs as a consequence of its capacity.[24]

[22] Herrnstein 1979 and Herrnstein, et al. 1976.   [23] Davidson 1999: 8.
[24] Allen 1999: 37.

While there is a lot of empirical evidence to suggest that animals are capable of discriminating, there is less evidence of error discrimination and correction, but there is some. Stories from Irene Pepperberg's work with Alex and Griffin, two African Gray Parrots, are suggestive, if not definitive. The parrots learned to speak English and with that skill were taught to associate specific words with objects and to describe various features of the objects, such as the color, shape, and material from which the object is made. When Alex and Griffin were shown two squares made of wood, one of which is blue and the other yellow, and were asked what is the same, they would answer "shape," and when asked what is different they would say "color." According to a report in 2000, occasionally when the parrots were tested the student research assistant made a mistake and would "scold Alex with a 'No!' when he had in fact given the correct answer. When this occurred, Alex tended to stick to his guns and repeat the right answer. Eventually the examiner came to her senses, and Alex got the reward he deserves." The birds were also observed correcting each other, and in a charming incident "caught on videotape, Griffin, while trying to say 'paper,' splutters 'ay-uhr.' Alex, seemingly pushed to the limits of his patience, peremptorily orders Griffin to 'Talk clearly!'"[25] This scene may suggest that Alex is not only able to distinguish between objects, but can also understand what a word is supposed to sound like and when it is incorrectly uttered.

There is more than just anecdotal evidence for correction of errors in other animals. Heidi Lyn, while analyzing a decade's worth of data acquired from working with two language-using bonobos, Kanzi and Panbanisha, has also reported on self-correction. She notes that "the apes frequently self-corrected when an error was made (self-correction was noted by the individual experimenters when the ape selected the correct lexigram after an error was made, but before any feedback was given by the experimenter). Kanzi self corrected on 89/1,070 errors (8%) and Panbanisha on 49/428 errors (11%), indicating acknowledgement of errors."[26] In another experiment conducted with orangutans to try to determine whether they were making choices based on their own assessment of whether or not they remembered where a grape (a very high value food item) was hidden, researchers observed that "one orangutan successfully avoided the test in which she would likely err."[27] Nothing bad happens to the orangutans when they make a mistake, so this

[25] Caldwell 2000.   [26] Lyn 2007.   [27] Suda-King 2008.

study seems to suggest that the individual is aware of errors and acts to avoid making them, perhaps satisfying Allen's (ii) and (iii).

Even if we come to accept that other animals do possess concepts, or that we would not be mistaken to attribute concepts to them, it is not clear that any other animal possesses as complicated a set of concepts as those that constitute a conception of the good life and can, therefore, be thought to be autonomous in this more robust sense. But before we deny that any but the most cognitively sophisticated beings can be considered autonomous, it is important to evaluate other accounts of autonomy, and there are many in the philosophical literature. We won't have to review all of them, but we'll identify some that might help us to determine whether captivity, even idealized captivity, violates an animal's liberty.

Self-rule

Autonomy is often thought of as involving the capacity to rule oneself.[28] Indeed, the word originally comes from the Greek "auto" or self and "nomos" or rule. There are at least two different conceptions of what it means to be self-legislating, as it were. One, coming from the Kantian ethical tradition, entails having a capacity to reflect on one's motives for action and determine whether they can be willed to be universal. This is a conception that requires advanced cognitive capacities, to be sure, and, as we just discussed, it isn't clear that any non-human animals have these capacities.

But all sorts of animals make choices about what to do, when to do it, and who to do it with. Many animals make plans, by making and saving tools for future use or by caching food to collect at a later time, as we've discussed in previous chapters. Social animals often engage in manipulation or deception to try to get what they want and to prevent others from getting it. So it certainly seems like these sorts of behaviors could be considered autonomous in the sense that animals are controlling what they do. They aren't being controlled. Another way we might understand what it means to be autonomous is to follow one's own wants and desires, interests and dreams, and not simply those that are imposed from the outside, or those which are internal but outside of control, like addictions. When one is autonomous in this sense, one thinks and acts and makes choices – one is an agent. There is a

---

[28] For a discussion of various conceptions of autonomy see Christman 2009.

sense of both independence and authenticity that is associated with agential autonomy. The dolphins and the hippos that we discussed at the beginning of Chapters 1 and 2, the wild vervet monkeys we discussed at the beginning of Chapter 4, and Jenny the elephant mentioned above, all seem to be exhibiting distinctively independent and authentic behaviors. Even when there are some constraints on choice, as there was in Jenny's case, she made her desire to be with Shirley clear, and it was also clear that she was not willing to succumb readily to the constraints she was facing.

To act autonomously does not require being completely free from constraints. Feminist philosophers, in their criticisms of the individualistic and overly rationalistic focus of some accounts of autonomy, have highlighted the ways that external forces or constraints are always present and even influence how one comes to shape one's desires and interests. Some of those constraints are often valuable as well, so they can't and shouldn't be completely ruled out. In the case of humans, the autonomous individual does not slavishly follow the dictates of family, religion, and the larger social institutions, nor does she always buck those norms. She can determine how to act in light of social pressures and expectations, and, in that determination, she expresses her "relational autonomy."[29] Individuals will be better or worse at exercising their autonomy. Some of that variation will depend on personality, temperament, and upbringing; some of that variation will depend on the types of interests one has; and some of the variation will depend on what is possible for that individual. As Diana Meyers has argued, autonomy should be thought of as a competency that is developed in "an ongoing and improvisational process of exercising self-discovery, self-definition, and self-direction skills."[30] Recognizing the ways that independence and authenticity emerge in particular social contexts expands the domain of those who are autonomous, particularly those who have been significantly constrained by oppressive social practices. The feminist conceptions of relational autonomy may be helpful for understanding whether other animals can be said to be autonomous.

By thinking of relational contexts in an expansive, ecological way, we can acknowledge that most other animals are self-directed, can adapt to changing

[29] "Relational autonomy" is an umbrella term for a variety of types of autonomous expression. See Mackenzie & Stoljar 2000.

[30] Meyers 2000.

circumstances, make choices and resist changes if that is what they decide, and improve their environments, often through collective action. Other animals learn from conspecifics and modify what they learn to suit themselves and their needs. They pursue activities that presumably they find rewarding. Not all animals in a social group do exactly the same things, eat exactly the same things, or spend time with the same individuals. They are making independent choices within the context of their biological and physical capabilities. There are species-typical behavioral repertoires that we might think of as constraining an individual's expression of agency, yet all of the behaviors within these repertoires are not fixed or determined. They are constrained both by what is possible and what is accepted by the social group, but there are all sorts of behaviors that can be said to emerge autonomously. Chimpanzees groom each other, this is a species-typical behavior. Who gets groomed, when, and under what conditions is something that an individual chimpanzee will autonomously choose. Some species-typical behaviors involve lengthy migrations, but who leads the migration, when the migration begins, and where the group is heading will vary. Some species-typical behaviors involve remaining with one's natal group for life and some involve leaving as soon as one is able, but the exact time one leaves, where he or she goes, and with whom, are choices that an individual makes, influenced by the community.

If other animals can be thought to be autonomous agents, then it makes sense to say that their liberty to act in the ways that they choose within their species-typical behavioral repertoires is valuable as such. Denying them the freedom to exercise their autonomy, to express their agency, by keeping them in captivity would thus be wrong.

In response, it might be argued that the lives of animals do not necessarily go worse for them when they are denied the ability to make choices or to pursue species-typical behaviors, in the way that the lives of humans go worse for us when our autonomy is not respected. Since many animals live longer lives in captivity, it might be suggested that their lives, in fact, go better for them when their liberty is denied. Leaving them alone to act autonomously, in some cases, may actually make their lives worse. For example, pursuing species-typical behaviors like territorial displays often leads to injuries and even death. There are many examples of animals in their wild state freely choosing to engage in behaviors that will lead to their own pain and suffering. (In the next chapter, we will examine some of the interesting suggestions that philosophers have made about whether we have obligations to prevent that suffering.) Humans also engage in self-destructive behaviors that lead to their own pain and suffering. Adrenalin junkies jump out of airplanes with parachutes that may fail, off cliffs with gliders that may crash, or off bridges with bungee cords that may break. Many people take on jobs that are dangerous, enter into relationships that are dangerous, or pursue activities that will, in all likelihood, lead to disappointment, frustration, and demise. We generally find it objectionable when the state or others act paternalistically in order to prevent individuals from doing what they want to do, even if it causes them injury. It is a violation of their intrinsic interest in liberty. Preventing injury or death to a human or non-human who may suffer as a result of her autonomous actions is, other things being equal, not a justification for denying her all of her freedom.[31]

Wild dignity

There is another, related reason to object to even the idealized form of captivity we are trying to imagine. When animals are kept captive, they are denied what I will call their "Wild dignity." Before we discuss Wild dignity we need to figure out how it differs from other accounts of dignity, and there are three other accounts that are instructive to explore. One is Kantian dignity, which is another way of speaking of the inherent worth of humanity. The second is what we might think of as Political dignity, a social or civic demand for recognition and respect. The third, alluded to by Martha Nussbaum in her recent work, is Animal dignity, which is grounded in each individual's species functioning.

For Kant, human rationality – the capacity to reflect on our desires and determine whether those desires can be judged to be a universal reason for action – is what elevates humans over other animals and what marks us as beings with unconditional worth or dignity. In light of the discussion in Chapters 1 and 2, we may ask why we should think of dignity as a property that all humans have, and we may wonder whether this is just another version of human exceptionalism. There are various scholarly answers to this question that aren't necessary to explore further here.[32] Instead, it is important to

---

[31] If the individual is unable to make non-injurious decisions, either because they are not yet matured or because of some psychological or brain disorder, then we may be justified in institutionalizing that individual "for her own good."

[32] See, for example, Shapiro 1999 and Sensen 2009.

make clear that the idea of Kantian dignity posits that there is a property that
inheres in humanity, and it is in virtue of that property that we recognize
and respect each other's dignity. Variations on Kantian dignity can be found
in some bioethics literature, where dignity is sometimes discussed not just
in terms of rationality but also in terms of other properties that we earlier
associated with personhood – properties such as self-consciousness, episodic
memory, the ability to communicate, etc.

Political dignity doesn't necessarily require that one accept that there
is a property or set of properties that all humanity has in virtue of which
we respect each other and recognize dignity. Rather, this account constructs
dignity as a way to promote human flourishing. The Preamble to the Universal
Declaration of Human Rights recognizes the dignity "of all members of the
human family," and that recognition "is the foundation of freedom, justice
and peace in the world." Political dignity, whether it rests on some inherent
property or not, ultimately can be understood as identifying a social value, like
justice and peace, that societies should strive to promote in order for members
of those societies to achieve well-being. We can think of Political dignity as
conducive to social harmony and human fulfillment. What is important about
this conception, and what makes it different from Kantian dignity, is that
Political dignity is embedded in social relations.

Traditionally, it is thought that only humans have dignity, that it wouldn't
make sense to apply the term to other animals. Of course, if we think of dignity
as being tied to personhood or the ability to construct universal political
rights, then this would be true. Yet, when viewing some forms of animal
captivity, it seems that there is something undignified about them. Consider
Suzanne Cataldi's description of her experience upon entering the Moscow
Circus. She writes:

> the bears in the lobby are made to look ridiculously foolish. Instead of chains
> or leashes, they sport brightly-colored clown collars – you know the kind I
> mean? – those thickly ruffled Elizabethan collars – around their necks. In
> their paws they clutch balloons, on a string. Bears with balloons may be
> comical, in fact I think they are, but there is something sad, something
> bordering on the obscene, about the effect of the collar. It makes me feel
> sorry, embarrassed for the bear. For the bear stripped of its natural nakedness,
> and dressed up like a clown. To be looked at and laughed at and photographed
> for tourists ... The animals become objects of fun, even of ridicule ... These
> bears are just the prelude, a sampling of what's to come. Moving into the ring,

to the actual circus bears, the act I remember most vividly is that of the "momma bear": a bear with a frilly pastel apron draped over its torso and tied around its waist – standing on its hind legs and pushing a toy baby carriage around the singular ring. The bear totters round and round the ring, lurching forward with the carriage. It seems to be on tippytoe, wobbling on imaginary high heels, trying not to fall. In striving to maintain its balance, the burly bear appears clumsy, klutzy – like a tipsy, overweight ballerina.[33]

As Rod Preece and Lorna Chamberlain note, "What matters beyond any cruelty is that the animals are portrayed entirely as something other than what they are ... they are compelled to act in a manner totally destructive of respect."[34] When animals are forced to be something other than what they are, we might say that they are being denied their Animal dignity. For Nussbaum, Animal dignity appears to be based on a set of species-specific properties that are part of what it means to be a bear, or a chimpanzee, or a parrot. So, Animal dignity is not unlike Kantian dignity, only it applies to more than just humans. The properties that are typical of proper species functioning, that allow an individual animal to live a characteristic life as a member of its species, should be respected. When an individual is denied the opportunity to behave in ways that befit their species, their dignity is being undermined. As Nussbaum writes, "there is waste and tragedy when a living creature has the innate, or 'basic,' capability for some functions that are evaluated as important and good, but never gets the opportunity to perform those functions ... it is not a life in keeping with the dignity of such creatures."[35] Similarly, when an individual is forced to perform functions involuntarily that aren't part of their behavioral repertoire, like holding balloons, walking on two legs, and pushing a baby carriage, their dignity is being violated.

There are a couple of problems with this account of Animal dignity, even though it goes some way to help explain what is objectionable about the Moscow Circus bears, as well as about keeping animals in captivity, even under idealized circumstances. One problem is with the idea of capacities being "innate." As we discussed in Chapter 2, it is difficult to identify what might be "innate," but, more importantly, even if we could articulate what we mean by a capacity being innate or a "natural function," that it is doesn't necessarily mean it ought to be valued. What is thought to be "natural" is not always good, and there may be learned capacities that are worthy of value and

[33] Cataldi 2002: 106.   [34] Preece & Chamberlain 1993: 206.   [35] Nussbaum 2004: 305.

that serve as a source of dignity. A second problem that can be raised with both Kantian dignity and Animal dignity is that the essential capacities – rationality for Kantian dignity and species functioning for Animal dignity – seem to be static properties to which dignity applies, but it might be argued that the capacity only becomes valuable when it is expressed and recognized as contributing to the well-being or flourishing of the individual. Individuals with dignity-evoking capacities exist in relation to others and within specific social contexts, and it is within those contexts that one expresses one's capacities and has them recognized. Dignity is sort of like fragility; we don't worry about the fragility of a delicate glass until someone who tends to be careless and a bit clumsy starts to drink out of it, and it looks like it will break.

This is why I prefer the notion of Wild dignity – it focuses on the context of expression as well as a dynamic, as opposed to essentialist, understanding of dignity. Wild dignity is closer to Political dignity but more expansive, as it includes other animals within their own social networks as evaluated through ours. Wild dignity is a relational notion, not unlike the sort of dignity that David Luban discusses in the human case. He suggests that "human dignity is not a metaphysical property of individual human beings, but rather a property of relations between human beings – between, so to speak, the dignifier and the dignified."[36] It may be helpful to think of the question of dignity as arising when there is a compromised relation – between the dignity violator and the dignity deserver. Elizabeth Anderson also suggests that we understand dignity as a relational concept, and she applies it to other animals, but she frames it in problematic anthropocentric terms. She states, "The dignity of an animal, whether human or nonhuman, is what is required to make it decent for human society, for the particular, species-specific ways in which humans relate to them."[37] I think Anderson's instinct is right that dignity only comes into play when non-humans are part of a social world in which questions of dignity arise. When animals are living in the wild, free from our interference, or at least mostly free from our interference, we might see their behavior as majestic or awesome and perhaps we might think of them as dignified, although the term seems odd in that context. When other animals become part of a human context, as they do when we hold them captive, their Wild dignity becomes a meaningful concept, because it is in these contexts where it is most likely violated. Making other animals "decent for human society"

36 Luban 2009: 214.   37 Anderson 2004: 283.

is precisely what it means to deny them their dignity. When we project our needs and tastes onto them, try to alter or change what they do, and when we prevent them from controlling their own lives, we deny them their Wild dignity. In contrast, we dignify the wildness of other animals when we respect their behaviors as meaningful to them and recognize that their lives are theirs to live. We may not like it that wild animals are aggressive, smell badly, throw or eat excrement, destroy plants, masturbate, or hump each other. Often, in captivity, animals are forced to stop doing the things that make them indecent to "human society" and made to do things that they don't ordinarily do (like pushing a baby carriage) because humans want them to. This is an exercise of domination, and it violates their Wild dignity, even if it doesn't cause any obvious suffering.

Companion animals

What about dressing dogs up in reindeer suits at Christmas time or putting cats in doll clothes? Can we violate the dignity of domestic animals the way we often violate the dignity of wild animals in captivity? Recently the *New York Times* ran a story about a competition for creatively grooming dogs. Dogs are sprayed with bright colors, "sculptured with gel, sprinkled in glitter and otherwise primped to Technicolor perfection." Sometimes the dogs are groomed to look like other animals – lions, ponies, camels, buffalo, sea horses. Sometimes they are designed to look like characters – the Mad Hatter, Elvis Presley, or angels. It takes up to six months to prepare the dogs, and up until the competition day, "dogs look like nature gone awry, as if they were groomed in the dark with blunt instruments and dipped into a box of melting Crayolas." The dogs' bodies are treated like canvases, and they are transformed into living paintings or sculptures or something in between. Some people have complained to contest organizers that this isn't good for the dogs, and one reaction from the master of ceremonies is, "All they know is that people are paying attention to them. They love it."[38] While it is true that most dogs like attention, this kind of attention – in a crowded room full of dogs being clipped and shaved, sprayed with dyes and paints that emit very strong odors – may not be the type that most dogs seek. Even if these dogs have

[38] Branch 2010.

been trained to enjoy this sort of handling, we might raise a question about whether the dog's dignity is being violated by being used in this way.

Domesticated animals can't be said to have the same Wild dignity that we recognize in captive animals taken from their natural settings, who have not been and presumably cannot be domesticated. Domesticated animals have been bred for hundreds of years to have traits that are particularly suited for living in human society. They are so different from their wild ancestors that it would be difficult to try to articulate what constitutes the Wild dignity of domesticated animals. Nonetheless, there is another argument that might be made about what is wrong with creative grooming and other forms of body modification in domestic animals. It is the same thing that is wrong with breeding dogs to be small enough to fit in handbags, creating dogs with hypoallergenic coats, breeding them to be prize fighters, hunters, racers, and guardians, and that is that we are reducing them to objects of use. They are tools or instruments that satisfy human desires.

That companion animals are commodities, having the status of property, has led some theorists to argue that even if all companion animals were treated well, keeping them is nonetheless objectionable. As Gary Francione writes:

> Domesticated animals are dependent on us for everything that is important in their lives: when and whether they eat or drink, when and where they sleep or relieve themselves, whether they get any affection or exercise, etc.... Domestic animals are neither a real or full part of our world or of the nonhuman world. They exist forever in a netherworld of vulnerability, dependent on us for everything and at risk of harm from an environment that they do not really understand. We have bred them to be compliant and servile, or to have characteristics that are actually harmful to them but are pleasing to us. We may make them happy in one sense, but the relationship can never be "natural" or "normal." They do not belong stuck in our world irrespective of how well we treat them.[39]

Because of the inescapable power imbalance in our relationships with domestic animals, keeping them captive is problematic. When humans bring non-human animals into our homes, the non-human animals are forced to conform to our rituals and practices. Cats and dogs are often denied full expression of their urges when their "owners" keep them indoors or put bells

[39] Francione 2008.

around cats' necks to thwart their hunting success or forbid dogs from digging or otherwise scavenging for food. While there are clear reasons that can be given for imposing such restrictions on companion animals, often for their own good, these practices have led some to object to holding domestic animals in captivity. The crux of the matter for critics of keeping "pets" is that no matter how well cared for companion animals may be, they are still property that can be disposed of at the "owners'" discretion.

While it would be a mistake to think that we don't control domestic animals, that we aren't in a relation of power over them, and that they aren't really our captives, these facts, in themselves, may not necessitate a complete rejection of sharing our lives with companion animals. All relationships, between humans, and between humans and non-humans, can be characterized as imbued with power dynamics. Power becomes problematic when it is occluded or abused. Many human relationships with companion animals are characterized by reciprocal care and attention. For some humans with physical, social, and/or cognitive disabilities, sharing their lives with, or even just spending time with, companion animals can make a profound difference in the quality of their lives. And the animal companions that attend to these individuals seem to enjoy and take pride in their work and the company. And even for those humans who are not disabled, living with non-human animals can be, and often is, a tremendously transformative experience, for both the humans and for the animals. As I have argued elsewhere, it is often in these relationships that one learns important lessons about developing ethical and emotional skills to address complexity across a variety of dimensions of difference.[40] When you have to figure out what a very different kind of being, who cannot speak, wants or needs, you must develop the capacity for empathy that can be very useful in other contexts, with humans and other animals. That there are important, perhaps unique, benefits that may arise from humans living with animals, however, does not eliminate the fact that the animals are captive and does not automatically make the relationship one that benefits the animals. Attending to and satisfying their needs and making their lives meaningful and fulfilling is necessary if keeping them captive is to be justified at all.

That living with animals can be meaningful and valuable for both captors and captives does not mean that having companion animals should be

---

[40] Cuomo & Gruen 1998.

a practice that continues indefinitely by allowing domesticated animals to reproduce. The issue of captive breeding is a vexed one in the case of domestic animals and in the case of wild captives, but for different reasons. Part of the value of living with other animals is that it provides us an opportunity to widen our perception of our own animality and of our place in the natural world, to attend to events and stimuli in different ways, and to develop empathy and compassion for beings that are different from ourselves. People who are privileged to experience the devotion and companionship of dogs or cats also tend to become more generous, patient, and forgiving. The animals should benefit too – by being well cared for, protected from injury and hardship, and by being loved. Since there are so many unwanted and uncared for domesticated animals around the world, there will be opportunities for inter-species living for some time to come. It seems clear that minimizing the number of unwanted animals by spaying and neutering will go a long way toward ending much needless suffering. When the global "pet overpopulation problem" appears to be solved, when domestic dogs and cats are on the verge of extinction, perhaps then we might consider whether completely ending "pet keeping" is an ethical requirement. Until then, we are obligated to provide our companion captives the best possible care.

Sanctuary

Indeed, providing all captive animals with the best possible care seems a straightforward ethical imperative. Since we have denied them their liberty, and in the case of wild animals often compromised their dignity, causing them unnecessary physical or psychological suffering due to our actions or omissions, without any obvious benefits to them, is clearly unacceptable. Given that we have taken them from conditions in which they could care for themselves and each other to conditions in which they are now under our control, at the very minimum, we have an obligation to prevent their suffering. However, this is not as easy, nor does it happen as often, as one might hope.

Wild animals are kept in financially precarious roadside attractions and unaccredited zoos, and, even before the money runs out, animals suffer in squalid conditions. Many wild animals are trained to perform in movies, commercials, and various sideshows and are warehoused in pathetic conditions until they are no longer commercially profitable. And there is a growing problem with "exotic" animals, who are bought as pets when they are young but cannot be kept when they mature. Some of these dangerous animals are released into parks and wetlands; others are kept but have their teeth removed or endure other bodily modifications; and they are rarely provided with social or environmental enrichment. Sanctuaries have been established around the world to address these and other problems arising for orphaned, abused, abandoned, sick, aging, or otherwise unwanted captive animals. The goals of true sanctuaries are to rehabilitate abused animals, nurture orphaned animals, provide companionship and enriched environments in which animals can express species-typical behaviors, and to respect each individual. Most sanctuaries are created to care for the specific needs of particular types of animals. For example, there are carnivore sanctuaries, primate sanctuaries, chimpanzee sanctuaries, and elephant sanctuaries, like the Tennessee sanctuary where Shirley lives. There are also sanctuaries for domestic animals – horse sanctuaries, farm animal sanctuaries, and, of course, dog and cat sanctuaries for those animals that are not adoptable. A number of sanctuaries have emerged in the countries in which wild animals are native, and their goal is to protect and nurture orphans in order to return them to their habitats eventually. The captives in these sanctuaries are just there temporarily, and we'll talk about the reasons why they need sanctuary in the next chapter. For most captive animals, however, sanctuary is their final stop, and while sanctuary usually provides rescue, there are some so-called sanctuaries that do nothing of the sort.

Many wild animal sanctuaries begin when a person who has bought a wild animal as a pet realizes that his situation is untenable. These people are often in a network of other exotic pet owners, and they provide a place for these others to put the animals when they can no longer be cared for in an individual's home. Some of the sanctuaries that began this way have developed high levels of captive care – incorporating the knowledge of professionals who understand the physical and behavioral needs of the animals, raising funds and creating endowments to care for the animals for their entire lives, and building adequate facilities to care for the animals' species-specific needs. Others have not taken such care, leading to what is now seen as a serious problem with "pseudo-sanctuaries" – places that, at best, think they are doing what is right for the animals, but lack the knowledge to do so, and, at worst, are commercially involved in exotic animal trade, but who dupe the public into thinking that they provide sanctuary for the animals. Some sanctuaries that begin with good intentions devolve into regrettable hoarding situations. In a study of fifty-six reported cases of animal hoarding, nine of those identified as hoarders described themselves as directors of sanctuaries and rescue groups. In four cases, the individuals were actually managing organizations, sometimes even animal rights organizations, with legitimate nonprofit status.[41] Hoarders amass animals and are unable to recognize illness, hunger, or dehydration. They are psychologically and ideologically incapable of recognizing that the care they provide is sub-standard. Often animals die in horrible states, and the hoarder still believes he or she is the best person to care for the animals. In one press report, under the headline "Animal Sanctuary Attacked as Spectacle," a hoarder was described as having "65 dogs, 20 wolves, a bear, a fox, a raccoon, and several horses and burros, all living in filth."[42] While there are a few organizations that seek to coordinate and provide standards for sanctuaries, these are voluntary, and there is no organization or oversight body that specifically regulates or monitors sanctuaries.

Some so-called sanctuaries are actually places where exotic animals are bred and sold as pets. This, of course, contributes to the captive animal problem. True sanctuaries are generally opposed to captive breeding. But this too has complex welfare implications and raises a challenge for those committed to providing the best captive care. The freedom to reproduce and to care for young is central in the development of important affiliative social skills that are necessary to build meaningful bonds with conspecifics and to enhance group stability. Denying captive animals the possibility to reproduce strips them of the chance to engage fully in species-typical behaviors, and this is particularly detrimental to females who are, in most species, primarily responsible for rearing young. Having infants born in captivity allows individuals to experience a full range of social relations, and it serves as enrichment for captive groups. Yet, allowing captive breeding perpetuates the wrongs that captivity poses. Elephant experts Joyce Poole and Petter Granli put the point vividly:

> Rooted in our knowledge of elephant social behavior it is our firm belief that it is not possible to meet fully the well-being of female elephants without the presence of calves. Yet we have strong misgivings concerning ethical issues surrounding the captive breeding of elephants and its longer term consequences. Any large facility holding a naturally functioning elephant

---

[41] Berry, et al. 2005.   [42] Arluke, et al. 2002.

population, complete with natural breeding and mortality, is likely to experience increasing numbers and, due to the confined nature of the exhibit, would have to intervene to maintain an appropriate population size. The issue of captive breeding is so problematic that most elephant welfare proponents argue for no breeding whatsoever.[43]

The same problems arise for great apes in captivity. Even those sanctuaries run by knowledgeable professionals who provide the very highest level of captive care – sanctuaries like Chimp Haven in Keithville, Louisiana that provides lifetime care for chimpanzees retired from medical research, entertainment, or no longer wanted as pets – cannot satisfy all the needs of captive animals, because they, like all reputable chimpanzee sanctuaries in North America, do not allow chimpanzees to reproduce.

Chimp Haven and genuine wild animal sanctuaries around the world are making a huge difference for captive animals. They rescue captive wild animals from conditions of deprivation and suffering and provide the animals with opportunities to make choices, to live with others of their kind, and to regain part of their Wild dignity. A common refrain in the sanctuary community is certainly true: "Saving one animal may not change the world, but for that one animal, the world will change forever." Yet, even when captive animals have their futures secured, are provided with access to the outdoors, have space to develop stable social relationships if they are social species, have ample opportunities to express species-typical behaviors, are not removed from their groups except when it is directly in the interest of that individual and the particular group to which he or she belongs, are provided with healthy and plentiful food in a way that is enriching, and are provided with opportunities to exercise and develop species-typical cognitive and behavioral skills, they remain captives.

And this returns us to the dilemma with which we started this chapter. Animals in captivity often suffer physically and psychologically, have their liberty interests frustrated, and have their Wild dignity violated. Releasing them to the wild may restore their liberty and dignity, but it will undoubtedly lead to tremendous suffering and probable death. Keeping them captive is wrong and releasing them from captivity is wrong: Is there an ethical way out of this dilemma? It is clear that creating conditions that minimize the physical and psychological suffering of captivity is an obvious imperative. This imperative

---

[43] Poole & Granli 2008.

will have serious implications for current captive practices. Many zoos would either have to close or fundamentally alter the way they conceive of their mission. Commercial animal enterprises – using exotic animals in entertainment or selling them as pets; circuses, roadside attractions, and horse racing; and animal breeding – would have to end. For some animals, such as marine mammals, elephants, long-lived birds, and perhaps monkeys and great apes, protected semi-wild sanctuary areas would have to be developed. In these areas, the animals will not be completely free; certain aspects of their lives, including prohibited reproduction, would be under human control, but their range of choices would be expanded and their Wild dignity restored. This would be an improvement, but it doesn't fully address the problems that keeping animals captive pose. There may be no ethical way to rectify the wrong we have done. Perhaps the best we can do is to attend more carefully and systematically to the needs of animals in captivity, to begin to put their basic interests ahead of our more frivolous ones, and to work to protect their natural habitats to minimize the need to bring more animals into captivity and, thus, avoid doing any further harm.

6   Animals in the wild

Ludmilla, known as Milla, was discovered as a tiny baby chained to the body of her dead mother at a meat market in Cameroon, Africa in the early 1970s. Milla was purchased and raised as a human child by a British couple who lived in Kenya. When the couple left Kenya, they gave Milla, who was then a toddler, to someone in Tanzania, where she became a barroom attraction at a local hotel. For years, she had the run of the hotel until she got older and bit someone, at which point she was confined to a cage, as so many chimpanzees all around Africa increasingly are. In 1990, Jane Goodall found Milla and wanted to provide her with a better life in the company of other chimpanzees. By this time, Milla was addicted to cigarettes and beer. Because she had never really known life other than with humans, there seemed to be no way successfully to introduce her to wild chimpanzees. So Goodall decided to fly Milla to a chimpanzee sanctuary in Zambia known as the Chimfunshi Wildlife Orphanage.

Most of the chimpanzees brought to Chimfunshi are infants, orphaned as a result of the bushmeat trade and the illegal smuggling of chimpanzees for pets and entertainment. Milla was nearly twenty years old and had been removed from the only life she had ever known, so her transition proved difficult, perhaps because in addition to her age she was one of the smartest and most demanding chimpanzees the orphanage had ever encountered. Fortunately, not long after arriving at Chimfunshi, Milla settled in and was introduced to her first chimpanzee friend, an adolescent male named Sandy. The two of them were eventually housed with other chimpanzees in a fourteen-acre, forested enclosure. Sandy turned out to be quite the escape artist, so eventually he was moved to a special escape-proof enclosure where he still lives with another escape artist, Cleo, and her daughter Chrissy, who is pictured on the cover of this book.[1]

[1] For an engaging discussion of the history of the Chimfunshi Wildlife Orphanage see Siddle 2002.

In the early 1900s, there were an estimated two million chimpanzees in twenty-five countries ranging from the west coast of Africa through central Africa to western Tanzania. By 1960, as their habitat became increasingly fragmented due to rapid deforestation, their population declined by half. Today, chimpanzees are considered an endangered species. There are an estimated 150,000 chimpanzees in twenty-one range countries. They have become extinct in four of the countries where they once lived, and their populations continue to decline throughout their original range.

The threats wild chimpanzees face are mutually reinforcing, making their continued survival precarious. The forests are being destroyed; chimpanzees are dying from disease, some of which are contracted from humans; and they are being hunted, trapped, and taken, usually dead but often alive, from their forest homes. Although there are legal restrictions on the export of live animals, the practice of trapping and shooting mothers and taking their infants for export for the entertainment industry and the pet trade continues to threaten chimpanzees, much as it did Milla and her mother. Since a chimpanzee is worth a minimum of $25,000 on the black market, it is unclear that the illegal trade will ever be curtailed fully.

Chimpanzee habitat destruction in Africa is the direct result of the exploding human population's need for more space and resources. Forests are cut to accommodate people, crops, and livestock. The forests are also being destroyed by foreign-owned timber companies who build roads into the forest, practice clear-cutting, and remove the tropical wood for sale overseas. The impact on chimpanzees and other forest animals is severe. As the forests shrink, the chimpanzee range decreases, which in turn minimizes available foods and puts chimpanzees into contact with other animals, including other chimpanzee communities which can lead to fatal conflicts. Some groups of chimpanzees may get cut off from other members of the community and become isolated in non-viable populations, as has happened in Bossou in Guinea, where only thirteen chimpanzees remain.

Another dangerous side effect of deforestation is that the remaining forests are now more accessible for bushmeat hunters. Bushmeat, or the meat from wild animals killed in the forests, poses what some consider the greatest threat to chimpanzees and other large mammals in the African forests, like duikers and elephants. The logging and mining roads have made access to the deeper parts of the forest easier for commercial hunters, who come in to slaughter mammals to bring to market.

Rural people living close to the forest eat bushmeat to survive. This sort of subsistence hunting for survival consists mostly of small animals that can be trapped. Occasionally, a chimpanzee will fall victim to subsistence hunters, but subsistence hunting does not pose a substantial threat to wild chimpanzees and other threatened populations. Commercial hunting is the real problem. To satisfy the exotic tastes of those in urban centers, the commercial bushmeat trade is decimating entire species. While the commercial trade provides economic opportunities for some in countries where there are limited means for earning money, the slaughter of chimpanzees, gorillas, bonobos, mandrills, forest elephants, and other large mammals is not sustainable.

An especially cruel by-product of the bushmeat trade is orphaned chimpanzees like Milla. Too small to be worth killing for their meat, baby chimps are sold to zoos or as pets, only to be killed or discarded when they get too big to control. Countless others are left simply to starve. Fortunately, there are sanctuaries across Africa, like Chimfunshi, where Milla, Sandy, Cleo, Chrissy, and 120 other chimpanzees now live. Ngamba Island Chimpanzee Sanctuary in Uganda, Sanaga-Yong Chimpanzee Rescue Center in Cameroon, Tacugama Chimpanzee Sanctuary in Sierra Leone, and Tchimpounga Chimpanzee Rehabilitation Centre in the Republic of Congo rehabilitate and provide caring protected havens for confiscated, orphaned, and discarded chimpanzees. Together with others involved in the Pan African Sanctuary Alliance, these sanctuaries are working to educate people about the bushmeat crisis and to establish protected habitats so that, eventually, some of the orphaned chimpanzees might be reintroduced into their wild environment.

In this chapter, we'll explore the perils that wild animals face and a number of conflicts that arise for animals in their native habitats. There are philosophical conflicts that emerge when we weigh individual animal well-being against the value of preserving species and their native habitats; there are ethical issues that emerge when we consider very practical conflicts between humans and animals, as well as conflicts between some animals and others. There are so many complexities associated with our impact on the global environment and the animals that depend on that environment remaining sustainable, that we will only be able to scratch the surface here. If nothing else, these complexities should remind us to be cautious and reflective in the face of daunting challenges.

Extinction

These days the word "extinction" fills one with concern. Five-year-old Josi, the daughter of one of my good friends, is very worried about extinction and whenever I see her, she promptly tells me about another species of animal that she has learned is "in danger." Although I was initially surprised to discover that children were learning so much about biodiversity loss and at relatively early ages, my surprise waned when I started looking at the available educational materials about threatened wild animals. There are websites, children's exercises, museum exhibitions, television programs, cartoons, even chocolate, geared toward raising awareness of the problem of endangered species. Of course, it isn't just children to whom information about the "biodiversity crisis" is directed. Unlike other environmental issues that we might directly affect by changing our diets, turning off lights, driving less, and generally reducing consumption, there is little an individual can do directly to save species from extinction. So, extra efforts to raise awareness are important in changing attitudes that ultimately can shape policy. Changes in public attitudes and a growing scientific consensus on biodiversity loss have led to some international attention to the plight of animals in the wild. But while there are important international organizations, such as the International Union for Conservation of Nature (IUCN), the World Wildlife Fund (WWF), and the United Nations Environment Program (UNEP), monitoring biodiversity loss and identifying species most in need of protection, as the Executive Secretary of the international Convention on Biological Diversity, Ahmed Djoghlaf, put it, "The news is not good."[2] In 1992, at the UN Conference on Environment and Development in Rio de Janeiro, popularly called the "Earth Summit," the Convention on Biological Diversity was introduced and signed by 168 nations. Signatory nations to the Convention committed themselves to reducing significantly the rate of biodiversity loss at global, regional, and national levels by 2010. Unfortunately, they have failed to meet that target. In fact, the rate of extinction is intensifying.

Although we don't know how many species there are, as most species have yet to be identified, scientists have estimated that species loss has reached an unprecedented rate. At the beginning of the 1900s, it was estimated that of all living things, including plants and animals, about one species became extinct

[2] "Global Biodiversity Outlook 3," available at www.cbd.int/GBO3.

each year. In the 1980s, that changed to one species extinction per day, and, by the year 2000, it is estimated that over 100 species become extinct every day.[3] Some scientists are warning that given the rate of biodiversity loss, we are in the midst of the sixth "mass extinction" in the earth's history – an extinction notably different from the previous five in that human activity is the cause of the current crisis. Indeed, whether directly, in the form of hunting, poaching, overfishing, agriculture, deforestation, other forms of habitat destruction, pollution, and wars, or more indirectly, by emitting greenhouse gases that have led to climate change or by introducing non-native, invasive species that compete with native species, we have had a heavy hand in threatening animals, plants, and entire ecosystems.[4]

The loss of "charismatic megafauna," though perhaps not always as ecologically devastating as the loss of other species, serves as a poignant reminder of just how damaging our behavior has been.

Recently, a Javan rhinoceros, one of the rarest large mammals on the planet, was found shot dead in Vietnam's Cat Tien National Park. It appeared that the rhino had been shot in the leg by poachers so that they could take his horn. Ground rhino horn is a valuable ingredient in traditional Chinese medicine and can cost thousands of dollars on the black market. It allegedly treats fever, rheumatism, gout, and other disorders.[5] However, researchers at the Chinese University of Hong Kong found that very large doses of rhino horn could slightly lower fever in rats, but the concentration of horn given by a traditional Chinese medicine specialist is much lower than doses used in those experiments. One researcher concluded by saying, "You'd do just as well chewing on your fingernails."[6] Conservation authorities have said there are only three to five Javan rhinos left in Vietnam and fewer than sixty left in Ujung Kulon National Park on the western tip of the island of Java, Indonesia. There is none in captivity. Historically, the Javan rhino ranged throughout Asia, but, primarily due to poaching, they are now extinct in Bangladesh, Cambodia, China, India, Malaysia, Myanmar, and Thailand. These are huge, long-lived animals that have no predators other than humans.

The smaller, two-horned Sumatran rhino is also critically endangered in Indonesia, with fewer than 250 animals in existence. Indonesia is, for now, home to the greatest number of threatened mammals.[7] Another grisly attack

---

[3] Myers 1979.   [4] Hails 2008.   [5] Van Minh 2010.

[6] www.pbs.org/wnet/nature/episodes/rhinoceros/rhino-horn-use-fact-vs-fiction/1178/.

[7] Vié, et al. 2009: 31.

was recently discovered, this time in Sumatra, where a gang of people poisoned a fifteen-year-old endangered Sumatran elephant, removed his tusks and chopped his body into bits before dumping it into a river.[8] There are approximately 2,500 elephants left in Indonesia, and the population is in decline. As their forest habitats are being destroyed for timber or converted into palm oil plantations, the endangered elephants and Sumatran tigers, of which there are an estimated 500 remaining, increasingly make their way into more residential areas in search of food. Conflicts between humans and animals are inevitable, and tigers and elephants are slaughtered.

The endangered orangutans of Indonesia are not faring any better. Found in the lush, but rapidly diminishing, rainforests on the islands of Borneo (where there may be approximately 10,000) and Sumatra (where there are an estimated 6,600), our great ape cousins are categorized by the Wildlife Conservation Society as "the rarest of the rare."[9] The IUCN estimates that their habitat has decreased by more than 80 percent in the past twenty years, and, if trends continue, this highly intelligent great ape may become extinct in the wild in the next fifteen years.

The baiji, or Yangtze River dolphin, was classified as extinct in 2007, after a well-equipped team of scientists from six nations traveled up and down the river and was unable to find a single dolphin. Using underwater microphones, they failed to pick up the distinctive baiji whistle, a sound that has "been on Earth for at least 20 million years" and will be heard no more.[10] The extinction of this freshwater dolphin was due to overfishing. Even though long-lined rolling hooks and electrofishing are illegal, they are still used. When the baiji got caught by one hook, the mammal would struggle and become entangled in the long line of hundreds of hooks, and eventually drown. The loss of the baiji was the first extinction of a large animal since the disappearance of the Caribbean monk seal in the 1950s.

Sadly, if trends continue, there will be many more mammals, large and small, to follow. Several primate species, rhinos and hippopotamuses, and cetaceans are currently listed as critically endangered. There are more reptiles, birds, and fish on the brink of extinction; various tortoises, bats, and many different toads and frogs are effectively extinct. While this may make for awkward conversations with future generations – imagine being asked by your grandchildren, "What was it like to be in a world that had elephants in

[8] Hasan 2010.   [9] Fearn 2010.   [10] Biello 2007.

it?" – have we lost something of value, beyond the individuals, when species no longer exist in the wild?

The value of species

When we think of a world without elephants, orangutans, rhinos, chimpanzees, or dolphins, we might very well think that world is less valuable than one in which these beings exist. If these species become extinct, it seems something valuable is lost forever. Of course, individual animals are gone and that seems tragic, but once an individual is dead she can no longer be harmed. When animals become extinct, there are no longer beings whose interests can be violated, who suffer at the hands of poachers, or whose well-being can be affected for good or for ill. Nonetheless, there is a fairly strong intuition that the death of the last chimpanzee is worse somehow than the death of Milla's mother. But articulating why that might be the case is difficult.

The perspective of attending to particular animals and their flourishing and the perspective of protecting species appear to focus on quite different things. For the most part, the theories of value that we have been exploring in this book recognize the value of individual lives, lives that go better or worse for that individual. We have discussed the importance of understanding the specific interests of individuals and how promoting those interests contributes to their well-being. We have been attending to animals in their particularity, trying to understand their interest in being free to exhibit behavior that is part of their species-typical repertoires, and exploring why preventing this behavior constitutes a violation of their autonomy or dignity. Of course, social animals rely upon their social relations that are valuable to them, so in focusing on individuals we have not ignored their social contexts. We have been looking at animals as individuals within their social networks as beings with distinct personalities, recognizing that understanding what is particular to each individual is one of the best ways to assess whether that animal is in pain, is distressed, or is flourishing. Our ethical attention has been directed toward individual dogs, chimpanzees, and pigs, not to the species *Canis familiaris*, *Pan troglodytes*, or *Sus scrofa*.

When we think about the extinction of the baiji and the near extinction of the Javan rhino, we might capture the value lost by focusing on the instrumental or contributory value of biodiversity. The existence of these species may contribute to a range of important biological, medical, genetic, and other scientific projects, and, when a species becomes extinct, we forego any possibility of learning more from that species and of enhancing our knowledge of the natural world. Species loss also serves as an indication of ecological instability. The loss of one species may do irreparable harm to other species within that ecological community. There may be a domino effect; when one species falls, others are in jeopardy. There are aesthetic values that are lost as well. In some cases, we are losing out on sublime, awe-inspiring experiences, whether direct experiences trekking in the wild, or, more likely, the experience of watching wild animals on videos shot in high definition. There is also the value of knowing, even if we never see them, that we share the planet with creatures that walked the earth or swam the oceans many millions of years ago, long before we humans arrived.

Recognizing the various ways that biodiversity contributes to valuable projects and experiences can go part of the way toward capturing what is lost when a species becomes extinct, but what about those species who we have already studied, so we don't lose out on learning about their genetic, medical, or scientific importance? Suppose we found that they aren't really that interesting scientifically, ecologically, or economically. What about ugly, annoying, or menacing species? Some theorists have suggested that the problem is that value theories focused on individuals cannot capture the intrinsic value of wholes, and in the absence of recognizing the intrinsic value of species, preservation of biodiversity will always depend on what is good for individual humans and other animals who might be harmed in some way by extinction. Unless we focus on the value of biodiversity as such, we will not be able to value all species threatened with extinction.

Some environmental philosophers have adopted a holist approach that locates value in ecological collectives.[11] J. Baird Callicott, for example, distinguishes between three general approaches to ethical problems – what he calls ethical humanism, humane moralism, and ethical holism. Humanism applies to individual human concerns; the humane approach extends our human-centered concerns to our treatment of all sentient beings, human and non-human; and holism, his preferred approach, takes the good of the ecosystem as a whole as a basic value.[12] He argues that human, humane,

[11] It isn't just environmental philosophers: there is a long tradition within political philosophy that focuses on collectives or communities rather than individuals.
[12] Callicott 1980.

and environmental concerns are quite distinct and that ethical theories that focus on the former two employ atomistic and reductionist arguments and diverge only in their assessment of what individuals to include in the scope of moral concern. Ethical holism, on the other hand, employs communitarian arguments that suggest that we cannot determine what is right or wrong, good or bad, outside of the communities in which those terms gain meaning. Ecological holism extends the community beyond humans to include species, the land, and whole ecosystems in its moral assessments of policies and practices. Ethical holism for Callicott is focused on preserving and protecting "the integrity, stability, and beauty" of an ecological community, and with the integrity and stability of the whole species as a locus of value we can see what is wrong with extinction. As Holmes Rolston writes, "Every extinction is a kind of superkilling. It kills forms (species), beyond individuals. It kills 'essences' beyond 'existences,' the 'soul' as well as the 'body.' It kills collectively, not just distributively. A duty to a species is more like being responsible to a cause than to a human."[13]

The value of species, on this account, is more than the sum of the welfare of individual members of the species. The species as a whole is valuable in itself. The holist view allows that the death of individual members of a species would be justified if those deaths led to the betterment of the species as a whole and, by extension, the preservation of the species. Again, on Rolston's view, "[p]redation on individual elk conserves and improves the species . . . when a wolf is tearing up an elk, the individual elk is in distress, but the species is in no distress. The species is being improved . . . deaths, always to the disadvantage to individuals, are a necessity for the species."[14] Though the elk and the wolf are not presently endangered, the point here is clear: an individual can be sacrificed for the good of the whole.

There are a number of problems with this holistic view, all of which needn't worry us here. But one of the obvious problems is that it seems that if a whole species was disrupting or threatening the integrity, stability, and beauty of an ecosystem, then the holists should support killing off that species, much as they support the wolf's killing the elk. (This may be particularly true if the species threatening the integrity, stability, and beauty of an ecosystem is a non-native species, which we will discuss below.) This is because, for the holist, there is a whole bigger and more valuable than the species – namely,

[13] Rolston 1988: 144.   [14] Ibid.: 147–8.

the ecosystem. When the two are in conflict, then, just as in the conflict between an individual's well-being and the improvement of the species the latter wins out, so too should the ecosystem win out over species. Further, in the ecological course of things, should a species be threatened within its ecosystem we should not interfere to protect the species, if extinction is what will promote the integrity of the ecosystem. Though the holist appears to be able to provide some justification for valuing species, the view doesn't provide any stronger claim to protecting endangered species than a view that recognizes the instrumental or contributory value of the species. An endangered species on this view is only valuable when it contributes to the good of the larger whole.

Holists, though attempting to recognize the intrinsic value of species or whole ecosystems, go wrong because they have a limited view of how to value nature. They seem to think we can value nature either instrumentally, which for them amounts to not valuing nature at all, or intrinsically, where value attaches either to individuals or to collectives. But nature can be valued in a variety of ways; it isn't that we are trapped in an either/or valuing situation – we can value both collectives and individuals; we can value things as means to ends (like money); we can value things as ultimate ends (much as we value our companions, partners, or children); and we can value things as neither ultimate ends nor mere means, but rather as constitutive of other things that we value (perhaps freedom of choice and privacy are such things).[15] Some values lie between means values and ends values and, while it makes ethical analysis tricky, that may be the most sensible way to address tricky conflicts. Ecofeminists Val Plumwood, Chris Cuomo, and Marti Kheel have suggested that traditional holists, such as Callicott and Rolston, present us with a false choice, and argue that we can understand holism in a less dichotomous, more comprehensive way.[16] Species have value that doesn't reduce simply to the cumulative well-being of each individual member of the species, but that value doesn't transcend the members either. There is value in the relations that the existence of the collective allows to be realized. As we have discussed in previous chapters, the well-being of most animals, particularly social animals, relies centrally on their ability to develop relations with others of their kind, to learn species-typical behaviors, to develop specific cultures, to

---

[15] I develop this idea further in Gruen 2002.
[16] Plumwood 1993, Cuomo 1998, and Kheel 2008.

communicate, to hunt, to play. Individual flourishing, in humans and other animals, crucially depends on a sustaining and sustainable context much larger than the individual, and perhaps therein lies the value of species. When a species becomes extinct, what are lost are the particular individuals and the whole community that allowed those individual lives to go well, when they did.

Before we leave the topic of why species matter and turn to the problems wild animals face prior to the point where they are on the verge of extinction, I want to return to the intuition with which we began this section. There does seem to be a strong intuition about killing an animal whose species is on the verge of extinction that makes the killing of that individual seem especially objectionable. I get distraught when I hear about any animal being killed to make some allegedly healing concoction to be sold for great sums of money on the black market, but I became incensed when I heard that one of maybe five remaining Javan rhinos in Vietnam was killed for his horn. Why might that be?

It may be because the Javan rhinos are rare, and we value rareness more than we value what is common. This is partially true, although it isn't obvious that we would similarly value a very rare species of mosquito, so it isn't just being rare that prompts our valuing. Jason Kawall has suggested that what is valuable is that the being in question is unusual, and we value what is unusual. A rare species of mosquito may not be considered unusual, as there are plenty of other types of mosquitoes around. Rhinos, elephants, and great apes are not only less common but have other attributes that command our attention. Kawall writes, "Valuing the unusual allows us to value species which are unlike most others, even if such species have large populations [so are not rare]. If we valued only population rarity we would have little grounds for protecting species until they became endangered. . . . we should notice that becoming rare in terms of population is also a way of becoming unusual."[17] So being unusual can capture the value of rarity, but needn't compel us to value everything that is rare, like mosquitoes and certain viruses. Javan rhinos are indeed unusual in all sorts of ways – they are rare, huge, visually arresting, and "extraordinary manifestations of survival."[18] And their unusual value can explain why their being killed evokes visceral condemnation.

[17] Kawall 1998.   [18] This is Rolston's phrase, Rolston 1994: 53.

Valuing what is unusual, instead of valuing what is rare, has another advantage. When a species becomes rare there is biological and ecological pressure to preserve the species, and often that pressure is used in the service of justifying the captivity of individual members of the rare species. As we discussed in the last chapter, there are a variety of ethical objections to captivity – animals suffer both physically and psychologically, and they have their interests in liberty frustrated and their Wild dignity violated. Often, arguments about the value of the rare species override the particular interests of individual members of that species. As Dale Jamieson asks, "Is it really better to confine a few hapless Mountain Gorillas in a zoo than to permit the species to become extinct? To most environmentalists the answer is obvious: the species must be preserved at all costs. But this smacks of sacrificing the lower-case gorilla for the upper-case Gorilla."[19] The individual becomes a vehicle for preserving the rare properties of the species. But valuing the unusual doesn't necessarily usher in the same imperative to preserve the species because that sort of valuing is necessarily contextual. Something is unusual in evolutionary, social, historical, and ecological contexts, and putting endangered animals into captivity may render them less unusual, precisely because you can go to the zoo to see one.[20] Valuing the unusual can allow us to recognize and appreciate something special about certain species without losing sight of the value of the individual lives of members of that species.

Conflicts between humans and wild animals

The extinctions we are currently witnessing are an extreme manifestation of conflicts between humans pursuing their interests and the very existence of other animals. Though animals who are critically endangered certainly deserve the international attention they receive, many less recognizable and, for now, more plentiful animals are also being threatened by human activities. As I mentioned above, habitat destruction as a result of deforestation, agricultural practices, mining and other extractive enterprises, as well as hunting and poaching, pose the greatest threats to wild animals, and all of these threats are economically motivated. Parts of the world in which wealth

---

[19] Jamieson 2002: 173.

[20] When animals are regularly seen, their status as endangered, and perhaps even their value, are obscured. Seeing chimpanzees on television and in advertisements has generated misperception about their endangered status. See Ross, et al. 2008.

and power are inequitably distributed, in which a growing number of people have little control over their life circumstances and few opportunities to make a decent living, and where governments are susceptible to corruption, are the most likely places where natural habitats are being destroyed, and, sadly, many of these very same places have high concentrations of biodiversity. In Indonesia, for example, a few wealthy, powerful families, together with government agencies looking to profit, control valuable timber concessions and allow the forests to be rapidly cut for timber sales and to create palm oil plantations. The elephants, orangutans, tigers, and many other forest-dwelling animals die as their homes are destroyed. Sometimes they are burned alive as they have no place to go when the forests are slashed and burned. In many parts of Africa, poor people, with limited options, clear land to grow food or use commercial logging roads to hunt bushmeat. In the forests of Virunga National Park in the Democratic Republic of Congo, around 200 endangered mountain gorillas, who surprisingly survived eastern Congo's violent wars, are at risk as their habitat is being destroyed in the illegal production of charcoal, called "makala." These are just a few stark examples of the conflict between human interests and the interests of other animals. The more drastic conflicts, like the assassination of gorillas by rebels to make a political point or the commercial bushmeat trade and the sale of wild animals for profit, which orphaned Milla and so many other chimpanzees, are already illegal, but the vast amount of habitat destruction is not.

In the face of such conflicts, we might initially be inclined to adopt a multifactor egalitarian approach in which we first identify the interests in conflict as basic, significant, or peripheral.[21] In order to determine the best course of action when the interests of two or more individuals conflict, basic interests must be respected above significant or peripheral interests, regardless of who has the interests. When the conflict of interests occurs over the same type of interests – the basic interests of one being conflict with the basic interests of another or the significant interests of one being conflict with the significant interests of another – other factors, such as the psychological capabilities of the beings or the context under which the conflict arises, play a role in determining the best outcome. In the cases we are addressing in which humans are trying (legally) to make a living versus animals trying to survive, we have basic interests in conflict, and if we were to base our determination

---

[21] Donald VanDeVeer developed a version of this view in VanDeVeer 1979.

of how to act on greater psychological capabilities, then it would look like the human interests would win out. While this solution is not speciesist, in that the like interests of the other animals are taken into account equally, it nonetheless is not a particularly sustainable solution for the humans or the animals, so the context needs to be considered and the conflict needs to be reframed. Depending on the specific situation, the conflict between these interests might actually be averted.

Environmental groups and animal protection organizations have called for boycotts of palm oil (an ingredient in virtually every processed food) and rainforest timber in attempts to try to bring the interests of the threatened animals to light. Non-governmental organizations are also providing certification for wood, palm oil, and other products that are sustainably produced which both educates and allows consumers to make environmentally friendly choices. Providing education and sustainable economic opportunities to local people has also had some success. In Rwanda's Parc National des Volcans, conservationists convinced poachers to become ecotourism guides, and, as a result, poaching has decreased.[22] Jane Goodall, who has probably done more to raise awareness of the plight of wild animals than anyone else on the planet, has adopted strategies for community-centered conservation. Her organization, the Jane Goodall Institute, has developed a number of ecotourism initiatives across Africa to promote "income-generating opportunities for rural populations while supporting conservation goals."[23] Ecotourism is also being promoted in Indonesia, Central and South America, and other places where forests and wildlife are in need of protection.

But while ecotourism may provide a short-term solution to bringing human interests in line with the interests of other animals, it is not without its problems.[24] The economic impacts of ecotourism are numerous and variable. One of the most important goals of ecotourism is the creation of jobs to provide options for local people to minimize unsustainable and damaging practices. But local economic benefits don't always accrue, because often an enclave economy is established in which local people bear costs but benefits are not returned to the local economy. Estimates of tourist spending that "leaks away" from host country economies can be as high as 90 percent from

---

[22] www.kent.ac.uk/news/stories/conservationistsdoubleachievement/2008.

[23] http://web.janegoodall.org/cc-livelihoods?quicktabs_1=0.

[24] Thanks to Brooke Duling for insights on these issues.

the Bahamas, 53 percent from Nepal and Zimbabwe, and 45 percent from Costa Rica.[25] Although the economic benefits of ecotourism are often overstated, the alternatives for host communities involve continued destruction of biodiversity, either directly or indirectly. And even if the economic benefits do not fully benefit local communities, there are positive environmental impacts, usually.

Not surprisingly, the environmental impacts of ecotourism also vary depending on the type and location of the ecotourism. Ecotourist accommodations can be problematic if they involve large-scale eco-lodges and eco-resorts, the impacts from which may include "crushing or clearance of vegetation; soil modifications; introduction of weeds and pathogens; water pollution from human waste, spent washing and cleaning water, engine fuel and oil residues, and cleaning products; air pollution from generator exhausts; noise from machinery, vehicles and voices; visual impacts; and disturbance to wildlife through all of the above, and through food scraps and litter, etc."[26] The long-term effects of these impacts on animals' social lives and well-being have not been well studied, but there have been some reports. Tourist disturbance has led to the collapse of the Galapagos land iguana's feeding and mating systems.[27] In the areas of the Sierra Nevada with heavy ski traffic, bears abandon their winter dens even if they contain cubs. Helicopter flights over the Grand Canyon have been shown to disrupt sheep. Disease transmission and stress have been noted as a growing concern with great ape tourism. Tourism can also habituate animals to human presence, making them less fearful of humans and thus at greater risk from poachers. A recently completed year-long study of the effects of ecotourism on gorillas in Bai Hokou in the Central African Republic found that the animals are dangerously stressed by tourists; the gorilla's feeding routines have been disrupted; and they have become more aggressive.[28]

Some have argued that ecotourism may be objectionable because it involves a type of stalking, understood as repeated unwanted intrusions, and in this case not always by the same person but rather by many over time. At best, this stalking causes discomfort and, at worst, leads to problems not unlike those observed in gorillas at Bai Hokou. Brett Mills, a media scholar, has raised the question of privacy in the filming of wildlife documentaries

[25] Lindberg 2001.   [26] Buckley 2001: 381.   [27] Edington & Edington 1986.
[28] Klailova, et al. 2010.

and asks whether secretly filming animals without their consent constitutes an ethical concern that wildlife filmmakers ought to be addressing. Of course, animals can't give the type of consent we ordinarily hope filmmakers obtain from human actors, but this does raise an interesting question in the context of ecotourism.[29] Perhaps there is something beyond the disruption and risk animals are exposed to from ecotourists – they are being denied their right, as Justice Brandeis described privacy, to be let alone.[30]

Ecotourism does not necessarily challenge the ethical understanding that led to the conflict between humans and other animals in the first place, and it is not often a force for addressing the underlying causes of poverty and disempowerment that are at the root of such conflicts. To the extent that ecotourism may perpetuate the idea that the wild places where animals live are entertainment destinations, it certainly should not be viewed as a panacea. However, it has clearly helped minimize some of the conflicts between the interests of humans and the interests of animals and is thus worth pursuing, under the right conditions, in some cases.

Another way to resolve the conflicts is by creating "preserves" or conservation areas specifically to protect wild animals and their habitats, and in these areas animals are mostly free from any human presence. The Goualougo Triangle Ape Project, a 150-square-mile section of lowland forest overlapping the Ndoki and Goualougo Rivers in the Republic of the Congo, was originally going to be an area off-limits to humans, but when it became apparent that the logging industry was planning to build roads and cut trees right up to the boundary of the preserve, David Morgan, of the Wildlife Conservation Society, teamed up with the Congolese government to be sure some humans were present to protect the area. Morgan, together with Crickette Sanz (a couple whose chimpanzee tool-use discoveries were mentioned in Chapter 1), is working to preserve a large enough area of chimpanzee and gorilla habitat to support long-term interbreeding populations. Most of the other chimpanzee and gorilla populations in other parts of Africa are too small or too isolated to support viable populations into the future. The project is also working with logging companies to encourage sustainable, reduced-impact logging.

Creating conservation preserves, when they can sustain a large enough population, has worked relatively well when the borders of the area are protected. For some preserves, where the population is too small, efforts are

---

[29] Mills 2010.   [30] Warren & Brandeis 1890.

being made to create "green corridors" that will allow the migration of animals from one area to another for breeding. One such project has begun in Guinea where primate researchers and the government are working together with local villagers to plant trees interspersed with sustainable food crops in a three-mile forest corridor to reestablish territorial migration between Bossou, where, as mentioned above, there are only thirteen chimpanzees, and the Nimba mountains, where there are many more chimpanzees. In Costa Rica, "jaguar corridors" have been designated to provide protection for the animals' migratory routes through areas that humans have developed. Humans are encouraged to avoid interfering with, or creating obstacles to, the jaguars' movement. A jaguar might devour "the occasional chicken, pig, or cow" along the way, but people, whose projects are in the corridor now, recognize that the animals cannot survive well in isolated preserves and that the long-term survival of wild animals is worth promoting.[31]

Conflicts between animals

Adjudicating conflicts between humans and other animals when the basic interests of both are at stake is not easy, but, fortunately, there are often ways to reframe the conflict so that humans can survive, perhaps even flourish, without having to destroy other animals. But what about the conflicts between animals that are, dare I say it, natural conflicts? The crocodile kills and eats the impala; the wolf rips apart the elk; the jaguar eats the random chicken, pig, or cow; and the Fongoli chimpanzees hunt and eat bushbabies. The impala, the elk, the chicken, and the bushbaby are all sentient, sensitive beings with their own lives to lead and interests that deserve respect. Of course, the crocodile, the wolf, the jaguar, and probably the chimpanzee aren't the sorts of beings that can ethically reflect on their actions. They are not moral agents, so we can't blame them for doing what they do. We don't judge what they are doing as morally wrong. But the lives of the animals they kill are worth protecting and their suffering while being killed could be prevented. Perhaps we, as moral agents, should intervene in predation.

The idea that those who argue that other animals deserve our ethical attention should be committed to ending predation is often brought up as a *reductio ad absurdum* to the very idea that we have ethical obligations to animals.

---

[31] Rosenthal 2010.

As Callicott writes, "Among the most disturbing implications drawn from conventional indiscriminate animal liberation/rights theory is that, were it possible for us to do so, we ought to protect innocent vegetarian animals from their carnivorous predators."[32] Is this right? Ought those who argue for extending ethical concern to animals protect prey animals from wild predators? Should humans ever interfere in predation? Let's imagine that a child is being chased down by a hungry lion. If the lion catches the child, then the child will be torn to bits and probably partially eaten alive. Let's imagine further that you are the only one nearby; you have a rifle; and you are a really good shot. It seems uncontroversial that you have a moral obligation to prevent this child's death. Now let's imagine the same scenario, only this time the lion is chasing a gazelle. Do you have an identical moral obligation to prevent the gazelle's death?[33] In both cases, there is a valuable life that will end in a horribly painful death. Since to say that one is obligated to prevent the death of the child and not obligated to prevent the death of the gazelle, because the child is a child and the gazelle is not, would be to invoke an unjustifiable species prejudice, it might seem that there is a moral obligation to prevent predation. Let's explore this issue from a variety of perspectives.

If we were to adopt a utilitarian perspective and assume that the child is too young to have the concept of continued existence, so would not yet be considered a person with a preference for continued living that would be frustrated if she were killed, and that the gazelle is also not a person, then there is nothing necessarily wrong with the fact that the child or the gazelle dies. What is wrong is the pain involved in the killing. Since utilitarians are generally concerned with minimizing pain, no matter who experiences it, other things being equal, it seems, at first gloss, like the utilitarian sharpshooter should painlessly kill the lion in both cases. In so doing, the sharpshooter will prevent this particular lion from causing pain to the child and pain to the gazelle and will also prevent this lion from causing pain ever again. If this conclusion is right, then it does seem we are on the verge of a *reductio*. Why should the utilitarian wait until predators are hunting? Wouldn't the best way to prevent pain and suffering be to exterminate predators painlessly?

---

[32] Callicott 1989: 57.

[33] Jennifer Everett sets up a similar case in Everett 2001: 51. Tom Regan uses the example of the lion and the child, and the lion and the wildebeest, rather than the gazelle in the preface to Regan 2004: xxxvi.

Utilitarians, in determining the right course of action, have to look at all the beings affected by an action, and, if all the predators were painlessly killed, the consequences for prey species would be problematic. Without predators, prey would overpopulate, leading to food shortages that would lead to slow death from starvation and greater conflict with humans as animals ventured into villages and farms to find food. These conflicts with humans will be less likely to have alternative solutions, and some of the prey animals would inevitably have to be killed. Killing the prey would minimize their suffering, but notice how the utilitarian is now committed to a cycle of painless killings – first of predators, now of prey. Perhaps prey species could be kept in preserves where their reproduction could be controlled. This would minimize their suffering, but at great expense, and it isn't obvious that the expense required to minimize the suffering of prey species wouldn't be better spent promoting greater good.

Perhaps a better way to go is to figure out how to minimize the pain prey experience when eaten by predators. Maybe utilitarians, rather than painlessly killing all predators, should train sharpshooters to travel the world looking for predators in the act of killing their prey and then quickly and painlessly kill the prey so that they don't suffer while being eaten by predators. This does indeed seem like an absurd solution. Again, not only is it expensive and clearly not the most utility promoting use of resources, but it is unlikely that successful intervention in most acts of predation would occur.

A utilitarian may believe a better world would be one in which the lion would lie down with the gazelle and painful predation would not occur, but recognizes that any attempt to bring about such a world would not actually maximize the well-being of all. It is probably true that our interference with predator–prey relations would lead to worse consequences than if we left well enough alone.

But, to return to our example of the lion hunting the child, should the utilitarian sharpshooter witnessing the scene let that act of predation happen? Most likely not, because if the lion were to succeed in that particular hunt, then it is possible that a pattern of hunting humans would develop and that would put the lions into more conflict with humans than they might otherwise face. In addition, the humans who lose the child will be distraught, and their despair needs to be taken into account in utilitarian deliberations. In their despair, they may set up their own hunting party and go out to find and kill the lion, maybe in revenge, or maybe to prevent further human loss, and that could lead to more suffering as well. Perhaps they will injure or kill more than just the lion who killed the child. These bad outcomes could be prevented if the lion was painlessly killed before catching the child. Notice that none of these possible outcomes would occur if the lion killed the gazelle, so there are non-speciesist reasons for killing the lion who is about to catch and eat the child and not killing the lion who is about to catch and eat the gazelle.

Those who are committed to animal rights may appear to face a problem when it comes to predation. In order to respect the rights of subjects-of-a-life, we are required to treat them in ways that are consistent with their rights and to assist when others are threatening their rights. But we should distinguish between humans threatening the rights of animals (cases in which moral agents are required to protect those rights) and other animals threatening animals (cases that don't constitute rights violations because predators cannot be said to act in ways that are disrespectful and in violation of the rights of prey). Tom Regan has suggested, in the case of the lion going after the child or the gazelle, that we have a prima facie reason to disrupt that act of predation if we can. He has us scare the lion away, rather than shooting the lion, because to shoot the lion would be to violate his rights. However, Regan writes:

> Our ruling obligation with regard to wild animals is to *let them be*, an obligation grounded in a recognition of their general competence to get on with the business of living, a competence that we find among members of both predator and prey species ... In short, we honor the competence of animals in the wild by permitting them to use their natural abilities, even in the face of their competing needs. As a general rule, they do not need help from us in their struggle for survival, and we do not fail to discharge our duty when we choose not to lend our assistance.[34]

We intervene with children because they are not competent in these ways. Paternalism is appropriate in the case of children, but not so in the case of individuals who are capable of exercising their freedom to live their lives in their own ways.

Gary Francione, another animal rights proponent, has argued that we actually do not have a duty to aid either humans or animals. In the case of the lion

---

[34] Regan 2004: xxxvii.

attacking the child, he thinks the child does not have a claim to aid, just as the gazelle does not have a claim to aid. According to Francione, the rights of animals consist of not being treated as a thing or as a resource for our use. He writes, "It does not necessarily mean that we have moral or legal obligations to render them aid or to intervene to prevent harm from coming to them."[35] In contrast, Jennifer Everett argues that there are duties based on beneficence that require us to aid rights holders in ways that are "respectful of that creature's nature, where this includes both characteristic facts about members of its kind and the traits it possesses as a unique individual." She argues that there is a prima facie duty to assist when an individual's flourishing is threatened, whether or not an injustice has occurred, but that flourishing has to be understood in the context of that particular creature's nature. In the case of wild animals, part of their nature is to live free from human interference, so respecting that nature entails not interfering.[36]

So it looks as though versions of both utilitarian theory and rights-based theories can avoid the *reductio* critics have raised. Feminist theorists, too, can avoid it. They argue that there are things to learn from the predator–prey relationship and caution against a type of epistemic hubris that plagues much ethical theory. In the case of predation, feminists would warn against interference, as we humans have a tendency to create problems when we intervene in the workings of the natural world. (We'll see vivid examples of this in the next section.) Witnessing predation is certainly disturbing, not for the faint of heart as they say, but there may be lessons to learn from the disturbance. Contrary to what paleontologist Christopher McGowan says, "The sight of a snake killing a mammal, a young defenseless one at that, may not be a pleasant one, but we should not view the scene with sentimental eyes. Predators have to kill to eat."[37] Sentimental eyes may reveal something that is worthy of reflection. When we witness acts of predation, usually on film, we are often prone to empathize with the prey struggling to be free from the grip of death, but we should also attempt to understand and empathize with the predator. Occasionally, the prey does break free, and we feel joy and relief, but we should also appreciate the struggle that the predator experiences. When Val Plumwood escaped the grip of a crocodile as I described at the beginning of Chapter 2, she recounts humbling and cautionary lessons she learned from being prey – "the need to acknowledge our own animality and

---

[35] Francione 2000: 185.   [36] Everett 2001: 54.   [37] McGowan 1997: 48–9.

ecological vulnerability...lessons largely lost to the technological culture that now dominates the earth. In my work as a philosopher, I see more and more reason to stress our failure to perceive this vulnerability, to realize how misguided we are to view ourselves as masters of a tamed and malleable nature."[38] It seems that the idea that humans might have an ethical obligation to interfere in conflicts between animals is based on a faulty sense of human agency, and it misperceives the independent value of wild relations.

Martha Nussbaum's capabilities account seems to be the only view that might recommend intervention, although it isn't quite clear. Nussbaum recognizes that inhibiting a lion's capacity to hunt would be frustrating and would not be consistent with the lion's flourishing. She writes, "a lion who is given no exercise for its predatory capacity appears to suffer greatly, and there is no chance that education or acculturation would remove this pain."[39] But she then argues that the pain and frustration might be minimized through strategies that simulate hunting. She cites the Bronx Zoo, where keepers provide a tiger with "a large ball on a rope whose resistance and weight symbolize the gazelle," as an example that she thinks satisfies the tiger and allows the zoo to forego providing the tiger with "a tender gazelle to crunch on." This form of enrichment certainly breaks up a boring existence for the tiger, but I would suggest that it is a bit of wishful thinking to imagine that playing with a ball would satisfy a tiger's predatory longings. Providing enrichment for captive animals, as I argued in the last chapter, is absolutely essential to help prevent physical and psychological harm, and it may prove a distraction from certain desires, but it doesn't eliminate those desires. When a cat is given a cloth mouse to play with, that can be entertaining and satisfying for the cat, but for many cats having a toy mouse doesn't eliminate their desire to hunt. Nussbaum acknowledges that we can't provide tigers in the wild with balls on ropes, but she is ambiguous about our obligation to police nature. She favors "intelligent, respectful paternalism" over neglect and is open to the possibility that humans may be able to intervene in ways less cruel than nature.[40] She is quite right to suggest that "humans are intervening in animals' lives all the time." However, the question should be, what form should that intervention take? When we consider below the form human intervention often takes, and the havoc it wreaks, we may want to leave predators alone.

---

[38] Plumwood 2000.   [39] Nussbaum 2006a: 370.

[40] For an interesting discussion of some of the conflicts within Nussbaum's approach see Cripps 2010.

Conflicts between native species and non-native species

The Galapagos Islands are famed for their vast number of interesting and unique species, including the blue-footed booby, a host of iguanas and tortoises, and thirteen species of tanagers, known as Darwin's finches. Darwin studied the animals on the islands while traveling on the HMS *Beagle* in 1835, and his findings contributed to the development of his theory of evolution by natural selection. Though native species thrived in the archipelago since Darwin's time, in the last quarter century, non-native species have threatened the existence of native plants and animals. The growing population of goats, brought over by pirates and whalers for food centuries ago, posed the greatest problem. The goats were eating the food that many species, including the giant tortoise, depended upon for survival. Eliminating the goats from the islands became one of the world's largest invasive species-eradication projects. $18 million was earmarked to kill over 140,000 feral goats in a five-year period on three of the islands – Isabela, Santiago, and Pinta. The goats were shot from helicopters; hunting dogs were brought in to track and kill the goats; and "Judas goats" carrying radio collars were released to detect holdouts who learned to fear the sound of helicopters. Those responsible for the eradication also created "Super Judases," sterilized females implanted with hormones to draw out males, who were then shot.

Though the goat eradication project is considered a measured success, and native animals have bounced back, so did other non-native species. Cats and rats are now a problem on the Galapagos Islands, and local human populations have reintroduced goats and donkeys. Tourism is also responsible for the introduction of a host of other non-native species. It is just a matter of time before additional eradication is needed. In an effort to protect native species, it seems that an endless cycle of destruction is required. The problems of protecting native species are complex, and this has led some to suggest a more comprehensive, less destructive solution to the problem that would study the possibilities of coexistence between native and non-native species, examine the xenophobia that may be at the heart of valuing native species over non-native ones, and prevent the massive slaughter of thousands of animals.[41] Some conservation biologists disagree and think that the value of native species always trumps the value of non-native species. And people concerned about the well-being of all animals, whether from Africa or Argentina, native

---

[41] Brown, et al. 2004. See also Jamieson 2008: ch. 6.

or non-native, object to the slaughter of so many, particularly when it involves pain, deception, and fear. But, as one biologist put it, "Animal rightists are a bunch of well-meaning pinheads who just don't understand."[42]

What should be done in these cases? As we've discussed in Chapter 2, we can't read ethics off of biology. That some species didn't naturally evolve in a particular location doesn't necessarily mean that species should be eliminated. Ecosystems and the species that make them up are always changing as well. In virtually all cases, humans are the direct cause of the invasion of non-native species, so perhaps it is our responsibility to correct our intrusion.

If a species is in danger as a result of human action, there are some who argue that we should do what we can to alter the course of the destruction. But this doesn't always work out so well. Consider the case of New Zealand, where for 80 million years the only mammals were three species of bats and eight species of seals and sea lions. When people arrived on the island, they brought mammals that forever changed New Zealand's environment. Europeans brought rabbits for both food and sport, and in just a few decades, escaped rabbits did what rabbits do and the population skyrocketed on both the North and South Islands. By the 1870s, rabbits had become a major pest, not unlike the vervet monkeys on St. Kitts discussed at the beginning of Chapter 4. The rabbits in New Zealand were damaging the natural environment by eating native plants faster than the plants could grow back. So it was decided that the exotic European rabbits needed to be eliminated to protect the native plants.

In the interest of doing what appeared to be natural, an eradication plan was developed that involved the introduction of the rabbits' natural predator, the stoat, a small predacious mammal in the same family as ferrets and weasels. Some argued that the introduction was an ecologically adapted way to control the rabbits; others worried that, instead of controlling the rabbits, the stoats would prey on native bird species, and they were particularly concerned about ground-dwelling bird species that were not adapted to mammalian predators. The latter worry was realized, and stoats have proven to be an utter disaster. Not only do they not control the rabbits, but they have also caused many species extinctions and are considered by the New Zealand Department of Conservation to be "public enemy number one."

---

[42] Krajick 2005: 1413.

Historically, our attempts to manage or control animals and nature have led to some significant disasters of which the New Zealand rabbit–stoat fiasco is but one. As our climate changes, there have been conversations about "assisted migrations" to essentially move species whose habitat is being destroyed to another, less-threatened, area. The success of the reintroduction of the gray wolf from Canada to parts of the Western US gives some conservation biologists hope. But there is also ambivalence. As one scientist put it, "Some days I think this is absolutely, positively something that has to be done and other days I think it's a terrible idea."[43] As new conflicts between humans and other animals and among animals emerge, perhaps we would do best to display more humility, to ask questions and explore options and to exercise restraint and perhaps even try to come to terms with tragedy, if need be. When it looks like animals are in great danger and we know we have an ethical obligation to them, it is challenging not to act. But it is also important to recognize that our actions often have problematic, unintended consequences, particularly when we attempt to intervene in the workings of the wild.

[43] Zimmer 2007.

7   Animal protection

Animal activists are known for going to outrageous lengths to get their messages heard. It would not be odd to see protesters dressed as rabbits outside companies that test their products on animals, or wearing nothing but lettuce leaves outside steakhouses. Some activists put themselves in cages in the parking lots of fast food joints, chain themselves to coffins to protest military experiments, or cover themselves in bloodied plastic wrap outside butcher shops. They have been known to stage mass die-ins in front of the meat section at grocery stores, throw fake blood at people wearing fur, and harangue circus goers as they enter or leave the big top. They use bullhorns; they chant; and they march. Well-funded activists run full-page ads in newspapers, put up billboards, or air television commercials. Sometimes they commit civil disobedience by participating in sit-ins or blocking entrances at sites where practices they reject occur, and they are carried off, limp bodied, to jail. Sometimes activists go further, breaking into laboratories or fur farms to liberate animals, destroy equipment, and otherwise cause economic damage.

As illegal direct actions involving costly property damage increased in the 1980s and 1990s, organizations that promote animal experimentation, agribusiness, the fur industry, and other "animal enterprises" pressured the US Congress to enact a law making it easier to prosecute those engaged in more extreme forms of protest. In 1992, the Animal Enterprise Protection Act was passed to defend any animal user from protests that involved traveling across state lines, using the mail, or using interstate commerce physically to disrupt, intentionally to steal from, to damage or cause loss of property to an animal enterprise, or to conspire to do so. There were a few legal actions taken against activists under the act, but one in particular captured global attention. In 2004, seven activists involved in Stop Huntingdon Animal Cruelty, or SHAC – an organization coordinating the US campaign against the international product-testing lab, Huntingdon Life Sciences – were charged with animal enterprise terrorism, interstate stalking, and conspiracy to use a telecommunications device to harass others. Much of the focus of the case against the activists was based on words on the SHAC website that included comments coordinating protests, reporting on what happened at protests, and posting the names, home addresses, and home phone numbers of those connected to Huntingdon as potential protest targets. The website stated, "We operate within the boundaries of the law, but recognize and support those who choose to operate outside the confines of the legal system." On certain occasions, the website coordinated electronic civil disobedience, whereby a large number of individuals would inundate Huntingdon and their affiliates' websites, email servers, or phone lines in an attempt to cause property damage and to disrupt business as usual. During these electronic campaigns of civil disobedience, the SHAC website also encouraged sending "black faxes" which used up the toner in the fax machines on the receiving end. The SHAC website clearly announced that electronic civil disobedience, like all forms of civil disobedience, involves breaking the law and cautioned would-be participants accordingly. Though electronic civil disobedience may not seem to rise to the level of terrorism, it allegedly caused Huntingdon's computer system to crash on two occasions and cost "$400,000 in lost business, $50,000 in staffing costs to repair the computer systems and bring them back online, and $15,000 in costs to replace computer equipment."[1] Six of the activists, who, along with one defendant later dropped from the case, became known as the SHAC 7, were convicted of conspiracy and internet stalking in 2006 and sentenced to between one and six years each in federal prisons.

The charges against the SHAC 7 were sweeping and the first time they heard about some of their alleged activities was through the testimony of prosecution witnesses in the courtroom. In a poignant statement made before giving himself up to serve his three-year sentence, one of the convicted "terrorists," Andy Stepanian, reflected on a few of the things he heard:

> Through testimony in this trial I learned about events and activities alleged to have been done in the name of animal liberation that disturbed me ... Though my co-defendants and I had no knowledge or connection to these events, I would like to make a personal apology ... Through testimony I learned about a man who was afraid to take his son to the park to see the dogs. No one should deny someone time with their child. To that individual

---

[1] Details of the case taken from the decision of the *United States Court of Appeals for the Third Court in US* v. *Fullmer 2009*. See also Cook 2006.

and his son I would like to say I am sorry. . . . Through testimony I learned of a woman who had her intimates posted and sold on eBay. There is no excuse for sexual threat, ever. I am ashamed that anyone would commit such an act. To that woman I would like to say I am sorry. . . . Through testimony I learned about people who were the focus of animal welfare protests, who had children with special needs like autism, who could have been potentially scared by the situations. No child should ever be scared. To those families I would like to say I am sorry.[2]

As protests continued against Huntingdon, the Federal Bureau of Investigation (FBI), with backing from various animal enterprises, continued its efforts to strengthen the Animal Enterprise Protection Act. Claiming that growing animal rights extremism was now considered "one of the most serious domestic terrorist threats" (along with "eco-terrorism" – extreme activism on behalf of the environment), the FBI convinced Congress of the need for greater powers to prosecute animal activism.[3] In 2006, the newly named Animal Enterprise Terrorism Act (AETA) was passed and now not only animal enterprises but those connected to an animal enterprise are protected. In addition to criminalizing property damage or conspiring to do damage, it is now a criminal act to protest in a way that puts "a person in reasonable fear of the death of, or serious bodily injury to that person, a member of the immediate family of that person, or a spouse or intimate partner of that person by a course of conduct involving threats, acts of vandalism, property damage, criminal trespass, harassment, or intimidation." Since the newly amended act became law, activists have been arrested under AETA for trespassing on the front yard of animal experimenters, while chanting slogans, accusing the resident of being a murderer, and screaming profanity; for participating in chalkings in front of the homes of researchers; for distributing flyers that read "We know where you live. We know where you work. We will never back down until you end your abuse"; and for using the internet to find information on researchers.[4] Some animal rights protests are certainly getting louder, scarier, and can be intimidating. Activists have taken to holding graphic signs, with gory pictures of animal abuse, outside experimenters' homes and they yell provocative slogans at neighbors and passers-by, sometimes

---

[2] From Andy Stepanian's statement to the court on Tuesday, September 19, 2006 in Wyse 2006.

[3] Lewis 2005.

[4] From "Defendant's Notice of Motion to Dismiss Indictment," Case No CR 09–263 RMW 2010, available at http://ccrjustice.org/ourcases/current-cases/u.s.-v.-buddenberg.

frightening children. In this respect their actions are not unlike anti-abortion protestors (except no one has been killed by an animal rights activist). Should these sorts of protests be considered "terrorism"?

There are many ways of understanding or defining terrorism, all of which are contested. Some definitions focus on the groups or individuals engaged in the act; some focus on those affected by the act. Most definitions include "causing terror or intimidation," but one isn't a terrorist simply by causing terror in others, as there are too many things that can be terrifying to a person, ranging from being a victim of a violent crime to being asked to answer a question in class when you haven't done the reading. The violent criminal is quite different from an intimidating professor, even though both can cause fear, even terror, and each is also quite different than a terrorist. Terrorism involves significant violence or credible threats of violence against persons or property and this violence or threat is aimed at innocent people (non-combatants) and is in pursuit of political, religious, or ideological goals. John Hadley has suggested that a component of "randomness" should also be included in an understanding of terrorism – part of what is terrifying about terrorism is that it can randomly happen at any time, to any one.[5]

Extreme animal activists engage in harassing, rude, and unwelcome protests; they sometimes threaten violence; and the clandestine groups, like the Animal Liberation Front (ALF), damage property. They do this for political or ideological reasons. The ALF is composed of loose-knit cells of individuals committed surreptitiously to causing financial loss to industries that exploit animals. The ALF claims they are non-violent and operate under the credo that "activists take all precautions not to harm any animal (human or otherwise)."[6] Whether it is right to call these acts terrorist acts or not, they are now classified as such under the AETA, as are public protests that involve intimidation. Given this new classification, the animal advocacy movement now can be said to have a "terrorist wing" and this has led to a tremendous amount of debate within the movement about appropriate tactics. As Hadley notes, "Law-abiding and otherwise peaceful supporters of animal rights may be tarred with the terrorism brush and come to the attention of law enforcement officials armed with draconian investigative powers hitherto reserved for people that commit mass murders."[7] And being so tarred may also cause

[5] Hadley 2009: 372.
[6] Animal Liberation Front website: www.animalliberationfront.com/ALFront/alf_credo.htm.
[7] Hadley 2009: 364.

those who might otherwise be supportive of the ethical claims of animals to dismiss the idea, essentially ignoring the message because the messenger is associated with those labeled as terrorists. There are significant consequences to having this sort of association, whether the terrorist label is appropriate or not.

Can the ends justify the means?

The animal protection movement is composed of a variety of different people and groups with very different sorts of commitments. There are some who are primarily concerned with caring for animals, either wild animals in sanctuaries or domestic animals in shelters; there are some who are working primarily on changing laws; there are some, like the SHAC 7, who are focused on shutting down a particular company; and there are some who are working to end specific cruel practices and industries – dog-fighting, or product-testing on animals, for example. The one thing that everyone has in common is the desire to change public attitudes and to create a more compassionate, just society in which the claims of other animals are recognized and respected. As we discussed in Chapter 1, recognizing other animals as deserving of ethical attention requires rejecting human exceptionalism which in turn will require people and corporations to make significant, time-consuming, and costly changes. Achieving these wide-reaching social changes will involve both personal and political struggle. As the late animal rights campaigner Henry Spira wrote:

> To fight successfully we need priorities, plans, effective organization, unity, imagination, tenacity and commitment. We need, too, to remember the words of Frederick Douglass, the black leader of the movement for the abolition of slavery: "If there is no struggle, there is no progress. Those who profess to favor freedom, and yet deprecate agitation, are people who want rain without thunder and lightning. They want the ocean without the roar of its many waters. Power concedes nothing without a demand. It never did and it never will."[8]

Within the animal protection movement there is disagreement about how much agitation and "roaring" is justified in order to bring about change. The

---

[8] Spira 1985: 208.

question of whether violence is ever justified has been the source of heated debate.

For some, like the ALF, who define violence only as the use of force against sentient beings to cause injury or death, their actions destroying property do not constitute violent acts. Property destruction causes economic injury but no physical injury, so it isn't violence. Others argue that intentions matter and that the ALF engages in property destruction with violent intentions. Consider the difference between accidently dropping a lovely vase and purposely picking it up and smashing it hard against the floor. In both cases, property has been damaged, but in the second case we might say that the property was damaged with angry or violent intentions. Is there anything objectionable about violently damaging property?

Those in the animal advocacy movement who oppose the use of all violence have suggested that being associated with violent action is counterproductive. Violence is not an effective means for changing public perceptions and attitudes. Some argue that it is inconsistent with the goals the advocates are ultimately trying to reach. In order to create a more just, respectful, compassionate society in which the interests of all are attended to and the conditions for promoting well-being for all are secured, behaviors and attitudes have to change. Replicating modes of action that are familiar and disrespectful will not move attitudes in a new direction. The violence that is being done against animals must stop, but fighting that violence with violence is a failure of imagination. As Wayne Pacelle, president of the Humane Society of the United States (HSUS), has said, "You do not topple billion-dollar industries by breaking a few windows. It may be psychologically satisfying to people who do it, and it may be true that at this time it doesn't feel like there are many options. I understand this sense of urgency and impatience, but I . . . think there's other ways we can get to a more compassionate society."[9]

While many in the animal advocacy movement reject violence against people and property, there seems to be widespread agreement that non-violent civil disobedience is permissible after other legal avenues for change are exhausted. As popular media tend toward covering spectacle, sometimes civil disobedience is the only way to bring attention to particular forms of animal suffering. However, in the US, this form of action can also be construed as "terrorism" under AETA if it leads to significant economic damage.

[9] Clyne 2005.

Non-violent civil disobedience can take a number of forms. Civil disobedience protests on behalf of animals usually involve trespassing or refusing to
disperse when so instructed by a legal authority. The practice of non-violent
civil disobedience is often associated with one of its most successful practition-
ers, Mahatma Gandhi, who used it to organize mass protests against racism
in South Africa and against British imperialism in India. Gandhi developed
the practice of "satyagraha" that, among other things, instructs against physically or verbally assaulting anyone, resisting anger in all forms, standing
one's ground, and accepting the consequences of one's actions. Though there
were spiritual components to Gandhi's form of civil disobedience, as well as
to Dr. Martin Luther King's, the secular ethical underpinnings are quite clear.
In order to gain respect for the message one is trying to communicate and
the injustice one is protesting, one has to give respect to those to whom the
message is directed. Physical violence and verbal assault are not respectful
acts. To gain respect and justice, one has to act justly and with respect. When
protesters stand their ground they are showing the strength and righteousness of their convictions. By being willing to accept the consequences, perhaps
by serving jail time or paying a fine for breaking a law, even a law that one
believes to be unjust, protesters are taking responsibility for their actions.
Respectful, righteous, responsible means can lead to respectful, righteous,
responsible ends.

One form of non-violent action involves "open rescues" in which activists
rescue sick or injured animals that are being held in conditions that are in
violation of anti-cruelty or animal welfare laws. Open rescuers also document
the violations and release videotapes of horrible conditions. Just as it would
be ethically objectionable to walk past a person in need of help, perhaps a
frail person who has fallen down or a child who is at risk of drowning in
a pool, so too, these activists argue, is it objectionable knowingly to allow
animals to suffer in factory farms, puppy mills, and laboratories. The practice
of open rescue originated in Australia, by the group Animal Liberation Victoria, led by Patty Mark. Open rescue workers, like fire fighters, emergency
medical technicians, and Red Cross volunteers, identify themselves and professionally provide assistance to animals in need of food, water, veterinary
attention, and comfort. Unlike reactions to the clandestine form of liberation, open rescues typically are met with positive reactions, probably because
no property is damaged and no one's identity is concealed. This form of civil
disobedience puts a human face on the activists' caring, life-saving efforts on

behalf of rescued animals and brings the plight of suffering animals to public attention.

Strategies for fighting speciesism

Activists are regularly seeking ways to convey the message that other animals matter – they are individuals with lives of their own to live; beings who can experience pleasures and pains, both physical and psychological; they are fellow creatures who deserve our moral attention. When we resist this message, we are, in a sense, resisting our responsibility and refusing to engage with a large part of the moral universe. When we act without compassion by ignoring the claims other animals make on us or deny that they call us to action because they are only animals, we are being speciesists, adopting a prejudicial view that, as we discussed in Chapter 2, is indefensible. All animal advocates are opposed to speciesism, but what should be done to combat speciesism in practice has been contested. Indeed, strategies for combating prejudice are debated even more often than forms of protest.

Pragmatism v. abolition

Early on in the animal advocacy movement there was a rift between "welfarists," those who are primarily concerned with ending cruelty to animals and developing humane methods of care and treatment, and "liberationists," who hold a position, often referred to as an animal rights position even when rights per se are not being sought, that is committed not to keeping animals in bigger cages, but to eliminating the cages altogether. Liberationists argue, much as I have been doing in this book, that animals are morally important beings who deserve our moral attention. Seeing animals as beings who make moral claims on us requires that we seek to understand and promote their well-being, not simply avoid cruelty. The liberationists are moved by the arguments against speciesism whereas welfarists are more or less committed speciesists but recognize that an animal's pain and suffering should be minimized.

As the animal advocacy movement grew, a new divide emerged among liberationists, this time about strategy rather than long-term goals. On the one hand, there are those who believe we ought to be focused on ending suffering and promoting well-being, sometimes derogatively called the "new welfarists." I will refer to them as pragmatists. Pragmatists are generally committed to ending the use of animals and want to minimize their suffering while that long-term goal is being sought. On the other hand, there are those who believe that the pursuit of reforms is inconsistent with the goal of ending the use of animals and that we ought, as a matter of strategy, to fight for that goal only. These are the abolitionists. There are often intense debates between these positions, as the abolitionists will speak out against pragmatist reforms. Abolitionist Gary Francione, who wants to rid the world of the use of animals for any purpose, including companionship, writes:

> our recognition that no human should be the property of others required that we *abolish* slavery and not merely *regulate* it to be more "humane," our recognition that animals have this one basic right [not to be property] would mean that we could no longer justify our institutional exploitation of animals for food, clothing, amusement, or experiments.[10]

Abolitionists cannot see that welfarist reforms can be consistent with liberationist ends. But pragmatists don't view an abolitionist end as necessarily in conflict with immediate welfare reforms. As Peter Singer has suggested:

> It's absurd to say that because we do one thing that is arguably bad for [animals] therefore it doesn't matter what else we do to them and can just treat them as things. You might as well have said in the debate about slavery that we shouldn't have had laws to prevent masters beating their slaves because as long as they are slaves they are just things and you might as well beat them as much as you like [until slavery has ended].[11]

For abolitionists like Francione and Tom Regan, the means of getting to the shared goal of ending speciesism and creating a society in which other animals receive the ethical attention they deserve, matters. They believe we should not "tacitly violate the rights of some animals today in the hopes of freeing others tomorrow."[12] For the pragmatists, who recognize that the ultimate goal is presently far out of reach, allowing billions of animals to suffer horribly and die while waiting for an end to all animal suffering would be an endorsement of far too much needless suffering.

Sometimes the disagreements between abolitionists and pragmatists seem rhetorical, but in practical terms these positions lead to different sorts of

---

[10] Francione 2000: xxix. See also Francione 1996.   [11] Leider 2006.
[12] Regan 2001: 144.

assessments of the problems non-human animals face and how best to address those problems.

One of the most contentious current issues is that of reforming the factory farm system. The HSUS, working with Farm Sanctuary and various local animal protection organizations, began introducing ballot initiatives in states that allow such measures, with the goal of criminalizing some of the most disturbing forms of animal confinement. In a resounding victory in California in 2008, the ballot measure known as Proposition 2, called the "Prevention of Farm Animal Cruelty Act," passed by nearly a two to one majority. Proposition 2 requires producers to allow animals to stand up, lie down, turn around, and fully extend their limbs. It bans sowing crates, veal crates, and battery cages. As we discussed in Chapter 3, these confinement systems lead to pain, injury, and frustration. The battery system of egg production is particularly exploitative and painful for hens. They are kept in small cages with six to eight other birds, none of whom can stretch a wing, and they are surrounded by tens of thousands of other hens also in small cages stacked in rows in large, ammonia-filled, dark sheds. In response to the awful reality these hens are forced to endure, voters in California passed a law that will require egg producers to switch to "cage-free" systems by 2015.

These cage-free systems take hens out of cages, but still keep thousands of them crammed in large, ammonia-filled dark sheds. The hens are still debeaked – the painful process that involves using a hot blade to cut through the complex horn, bone, and sensitive tissue of the hen's beak. As we've discussed, this procedure leads to deformities that prevent hens from eating, drinking, or preening normally. Industrial egg production requires that male chicks be killed when they are hatched, and cage-free hens, like their battery-caged sisters, are sent to slaughter after a year. Sometimes cage-free hens can go outside of the shed, but the exits are very small and the sheds so crowded that only the hens closest to the doors can get out, and, because hens like to be with other hens, very few of those who have the opportunity to go outside do so.

There is no question that the move from the battery-cage system of egg production to the cage-free system represents an improvement in the welfare of the hens, albeit a rather small improvement. The improvement for sows and calves are similarly small. But, so many hens, pigs, and calves suffer so horribly that improving the conditions even minimally amounts to a vast overall improvement in the amount of suffering, given that people are still eating eggs and pork and veal. Imagine there is a pill that will reduce your migraine to a headache. Your head would still hurt and being rid of all pain would be ideal, but chances are you would want to take the pill because a headache is better than a migraine. Abolitionists would, figuratively, deny you the pill. For those opposed to any use of animals, cage-free systems of egg production work to prolong the violation of the rights of these animals as it makes people feel better about their abuse. Abolitionists point out that many people conflate "cage-free" with "cruelty-free" and they worry about the complacency that these small improvements encourage. Some abolitionists argue that creating more humane conditions while still using animals is essentially an endorsement of consuming animals and they fear that the number of animals used will increase rather than decrease as a result. While rarely admitting it publicly, many abolitionists think the chance of actually ending the use of animals is greater if the conditions in which they exist are worse. Francione publicly urged animal advocates to vote against Proposition 2, claiming that the only ethically sound way to address animal exploitation is to devote all resources to non-violent vegan education programs.

Interestingly, the campaign that led to the passage of Proposition 2 might be considered one of the most successful non-violent animal advocacy and education campaigns ever conducted. Eight million people voted in favor of Proposition 2, more than any citizen initiative in state history.[13] But, millions more witnessed the cruel practices of agribusiness during the campaign. Since the passage of Proposition 2, the California legislature has strengthened a range of animal protection laws. More people are actively interested in vegetarian and vegan lifestyles; schools in parts of California have instituted "Meat Free Mondays"; and restaurants see the use of cage-free eggs as good for business. A recent study of the effects Proposition 2 has had on egg-buying habits, for example, suggests "that the very act of putting an issue like Prop 2 on the ballot affects consumers' preferences – likely because consumers are largely unaware of and have incorrect beliefs about modern agricultural practices."[14] Research done in the Bay Area shows that in response to news stories about Proposition 2, demand for cage-free eggs increased 180 percent, despite higher prices, and demand for cheaper battery-cage eggs in retail markets dropped. California activists have reported that there have been more volunteers for a range of animal protection campaigns after Proposition 2

[13] Cone 2009.   [14] Lusk 2010: 15–16.

passed than before and there is a great feeling of optimism among activists, which is a welcome change. As California Senator Dean Florez said, "Prop. 2 didn't just do something to egg processors, it changed a thought process."[15] Indeed it has, as *New York Times* columnist (and meat-eater) Nicholas Kristof commented after the passage of Proposition 2, "What we're seeing now is an interesting moral moment: a grass-roots effort by members of one species to promote the welfare of another" and this marks a "profound difference from past centuries: animal rights are now firmly on the mainstream ethical agenda."[16]

Two lessons can be learned from this extraordinarily successful reform effort: incremental changes can be helpful in ending the immediate suffering of actual animals while industrial exploitation inevitably continues and these reform campaigns have consequences that reach beyond reducing animal suffering. Both abolitionists and pragmatists can ultimately argue against egg consumption, but in the time it takes for people to change what they eat hens will suffer less than they would have if Proposition 2 did not pass. We can't know exactly how each Californian's diet, attitude, and other behavior changed after Proposition 2 (we don't know how many people have given up eating animal products, for example). But we have many good reasons to believe that the claims animals make on us are being heard by more people than before the campaign began.

Single-issue campaigns v. anti-oppression alliances

It might seem that the abolitionist claim that vegan education is the only ethically defensible strategy to combat speciesism is a bit single-minded. When they encourage veganism, however, the abolitionists go beyond diet. Veganism rejects all forms of animal exploitation. So some of the abolitionists argue that they are not calling for single-issue campaigning: they are opposed to all animal uses – for food, in laboratories, in zoos, circuses, and for other forms of human entertainment. The abolitionists cannot support a campaign to end the use of elephants in circuses, for example, because that might be construed as accepting the use of other animals in circuses or elephants and other animals in zoos and aquariums. A campaign to retire chimpanzees from biomedical research would be rejected by abolitionists because it may

---

[15] Cone 2009.   [16] Kristof 2009.

appear to endorse research on animals. To fight against the use of elephants in circuses, to retire chimpanzees from research laboratories, or to improve the conditions on factory farms is what abolitionists think of as single-issue campaign strategies, and since abolitionists are opposed to such strategies they imagine that they are against single-issue campaigns.

However, most social justice advocates have a broader vision of single-issue campaigning, by which they tend to mean only campaigning against one type of injustice, like speciesism, and not also attending to environmental issues, gender and racial justice, the problems of globalization, poverty, heterosexism, unequal access to the means to achieve well-being, etc. From the larger perspective of justice or anti-oppression activism, the abolitionists' call for non-violent vegan education campaigns is not all that different from the pragmatist call for bipartisanship in lobbying for animals. For example, Pacelle describes the mission of HSUS's lobbying organization as narrowly focused on "a legislator's or candidate's record on animal issues only." He says they will support democrats or republicans who are good on animal issues. This is what might be considered single-issue political campaigning.

Many years ago, I recounted an example of the potential problem of single-issue campaigning.[17] I had come across a group of feminist activists in New York's Grand Central Station who were collecting signatures for a petition to ban pornography. I was very interested in an image that these women were displaying at their table: it was a cover of *Hustler* magazine that depicted a woman's body being put through a meat grinder. It was a perfect example of what Carol Adams has since described as "the sexual politics of meat."[18] I told the activists that I was interested in the connections between the exploitation of women and the commodification of animals and was barraged with accusations challenging my feminist commitment. If I thought it appropriate to lower women to the status of animals, they had no interest in talking to me. Of course, I don't accept animals' lower status any more than I accept women's lower status. Rather, I was and am engaged in analyzing the connections between the way that women, people of color, and animals are seen as "others" – as beings that are viewed as resources or tools in the construction of the privilege associated with being white, human, and a man. This process of "othering" is a precondition for oppression as it aids in denying members of certain groups full moral consideration and agency because of their

[17] Gruen 1993.   [18] Adams 1990.

difference. Othering enables those in power to create moral distance which allows them to overlook or ignore their connections and obligations to those that deserve moral attention. Feminist theorists and activists have been laying the groundwork for understanding the working of sexism and racism, work that is helpful to rethinking the human–animal dualism. Unfortunately, the anti-pornography feminists are not alone in their dismissal of those interested in the connection between the oppression of woman and the oppression of animals, although awareness of these connections has grown since my jarring encounter in Grand Central.

One obstacle to getting feminists to take animal interests seriously is the regular use of sexist tactics in the highly publicized media campaigns of one of the largest animal advocacy groups, People for the Ethical Treatment of Animals (PETA). PETA is accused of commodifying women and sexuality by reinforcing harmful stereotypes in order to sell their animal rights message and often it isn't clear precisely what message they are selling – women look sexier if they don't eat meat or wear fur and men are better sexually or will get better sex from women if they don't eat meat? Sex, traditionally, sells, but, as some feminists have argued, the message of care, compassion, and justice gets lost in this particular exchange.[19] In a response to complaints about the offensiveness of some of their campaigns, PETA's website states: "PETA does make a point of having something for all tastes, from the most conservative to the most radical and from the most tasteless to the most refined."[20] And herein lies one of the problems with single-issue campaigns: the larger political context in which the messages are presented is being ignored. Everyone's "tastes," particularly those of the sexist, racist, or homophobe, should not be catered to simply because those people otherwise support animal rights. Attitudes of human exceptionalism, entitlement, and disrespect play a central role in the social rejection of the idea that other animals matter, just as attitudes of male superiority, entitlement, and disrespect play a central role in the perpetuation of sexism. Challenging those underlying attitudes in the case of women, and other traditionally disempowered peoples, may be a better strategy than perpetuating them, in the hopes of communicating a different way of thinking about the ethical attention that "others" deserve.

The most vocal animal advocates and the leading animal protection organizations, whether they are abolitionists or pragmatists, seem committed to

---

[19] Adams 2004.   [20] www.peta.org/campaigns/ar-petatactics.asp.

single-issue campaigning. Such campaigning has its value, particularly when it leads to the improvement of well-being for animals. But it is also important to be mindful of the connected structures of power that speciesism relies on and reinforces.[21] Understanding animal liberation in terms of oppression provides for an importantly different, and arguably deeper, analysis of not only our current practices toward non-human animals but also of the ways such practices support unjust and harmful social and political structures of power. For those who are prone to identify with and want to help the least well off or the weakest among us it will be important to try to see how oppression is operating in other contexts. For those who are fighting their own oppression, recognizing the way others, including other animals, are struggling cannot only provide insights into the working of the particular oppression being fought, but can also be the basis of building alliances. There may also be perceptual as well as practical advantages to engaging in a broad analysis of and collective resistance to oppression. The oppressive attitudes and practices that non-human animals are subject to are not unlike the oppressive practices that thwart the flourishing of marginalized groups. Understanding these practices as expressions of power and privilege, as well as of cruelty, ignorance, and complacency, may help activists to construct even more effective campaigns and to provide opportunities for building more successful alliances.

Importantly, as we know from situations of human oppression, there are often contexts in which conflicts between the interests of various groups require compromises in order to eliminate oppression. What is necessary, often, is identifying ways to attend respectfully to the needs, interests, and desires of the members of the oppressed groups on their own terms. But satisfying all of those needs, interests, and desires is not always possible. An absence of oppression does not always translate into either complete freedom or a life free from pain or distress, and the abolitionists as well as the pragmatists would do well to reflect on these political realities.

Ideas v. animals

Failure to attend to the political limitations one inevitably bumps up against when holding too tightly to an idea or set of ideas may hinder successful work

---

[21] Feminists who think about the oppression of animals as related to other oppression have done the most work here. For a general discussion see Gruen & Weil 2010. See also Gaard 1993, Donovan 1990, Donovan and Adams 2007, and Harper 2010.

to eliminate speciesism. Absolutist commitments and demands for purity are not just strategically ineffectual, but can also be self-defeating. Sometimes ideological commitments and the actions that flow from them can actually injure animals, violate their interests, and in some cases, even kill them.

I witnessed such a tragedy some years ago when one animal protection organization, with strong ideological commitments against any "use" of animals, was supporting an animal refuge that held hundreds of animals, including over sixty chimpanzees, and that was involved in a dispute with other animal protection organizations that were trying to improve the conditions at the refuge. This was an internecine conflict between animal protection groups and, as is often the case in such battles, the well-being of actual animals took a back seat. One of the main issues was that the refuge refused to provide enrichment for the primates because they were opposed, on principle, to human interference with wild animals. As we discussed in the last chapter, human interference with animals in the wild surely can have negative consequences. However, sometimes, as when logging companies or other extracting industries are threatening, a protective human presence may be warranted. In this case, however, we are talking about wild animals in captivity. The refuge apparently believed that simply providing food and water, but otherwise leaving wild animals more or less alone in captivity, constitutes respecting the animals. So, when this refuge received nine enculturated chimpanzees who had worked in cognition research and were raised to rely on humans to provide them with not just food and water but emotional and intellectual stimulation as well as help organizing their social structure, the refuge maintained its commitment to minimal human involvement to the detriment of the chimpanzees.

The chimpanzees' caregivers pleaded to be allowed to help them make the transition, but the refuge refused, in part because these individuals worked in a "lab," and thus were thought to support the "use" of chimpanzees. This "lab," which I visited a number of times, was less what you might imagine a laboratory to be and more like a daycare center. Though small, there were a number of indoor rooms with brightly painted walls, outdoor areas for the chimpanzees to nap in the sunshine, and the chimpanzees were provided with enrichment, fresh fruits, vegetables, nuts, and other treats. When they were interested, they could do work on a computer to match pictures to words or to count items. The chimpanzees willingly participated in the cognition studies because they received preferred treats, like grapes, when they did. The women who cared for the chimpanzees were dedicated to the well-being of each individual and also considered themselves to be animal advocates. Six of the chimpanzees came to this center as infants from labs where they would have undergone invasive medical experiments; at the center they were reared as human infants. One of the chimpanzees was rescued from a roadside attraction where he was chained; one of the chimpanzees came from a zoo; and one of the chimpanzees was retired from a more intense type of cognition research after thirty years. The transfer of these nine chimpanzees to the refuge was not something that anyone who knew or worked with these chimpanzees wanted to happen.

The refuge was not interested in facts about the needs and interests of these particular chimpanzees. They and their supporters believe "use is use" and, despite repeated pleading, they refused to allow the caregivers, who had volunteered their time and expertise, to help the chimpanzees. At the refuge the chimpanzees suffered from neglect – two of the older females stopped eating and two of the male chimpanzees died. Fortunately, before further tragedy could occur, state officials stepped in and the chimpanzees were moved to a facility that could provide for their specific needs.

Animal advocates and abolitionists who are opposed to "institutions of use" sometimes put that ideological commitment above the immediate well-being of individual animals and refuse to address conditions that will directly improve an animal's ability to flourish. As we discussed in Chapter 5, there is a dilemma about what to do with long-lived captive animals who cannot be returned to the wild, like chimpanzees. Captivity is not ideal, as we discussed, but it is inevitable for the 2,000 chimpanzees currently in captivity in the US. These chimpanzees live in conditions ranging from naturalistic, group enclosures, where the chimpanzees are given options about what to play with, what to eat, and who to spend time with, to sterile, solitary conditions in which everything they do is completely controlled by masked, gloved humans. For most captive chimpanzees, the conditions are somewhere in between. From a particular ideological perspective, these conditions are essentially equivalent in that they all represent a violation of the chimpanzees' rights to be free. But here the idea of freedom is at odds with the well-being of actual captive individual animals. Even though zoos are not, all things considered, ethically defensible, in practice some zoos may be the best place for captive chimpanzees to live meaningful, safe, comfortable lives. Insofar as activists are unwilling to discuss improving conditions of "slavery," it is unclear whether they have spent any time attending to actual animals at all.

Ideological purity and absolutist commitments can also be seen as alienating, elitist, and self-absorbed. As we discussed in Chapter 3, there are important contexts in which using other animals for food may be justified. This is the view that ecofeminists call "contextual moral vegetarianism," which allows that there are ways in which gender, class, race, ethnicity, and geographical location can create genuine difficulties with choosing a vegetarian diet. There are people living in arctic regions, for example, for whom a vegetarian diet does not make practical sense. And there are many people in the world for whom access to protein is limited, and often their very survival depends on killing animals. Sometimes the animals that are killed for food are chimpanzees and other endangered animals, as we discussed in the previous chapter. So it may be worth considering models of symbiotic living and respectful use that might allow for non-oppressive egg or milk consumption, for example.

Of course, ideas matter and acting ethically often means sticking to one's principles and ideological commitments however unpopular. But, in the face of the wide-ranging injustices that other animals confront and the corresponding complacency of most people, stridency may not do very much to promote the flourishing of all animals nor bring about desired ends.

Empathetic action

I began this book by exploring the deeply entrenched idea that humans are unique and better than other animals. I argued that the normative conclusion of human exceptionalism is prejudicial and thus cannot be supported, and I hope that by this point you have accepted that argument. What is also clear is that humans are indeed unique among animals. One thing that makes us so different comes to light in the debates between various animal protection advocates, and that is that we engage in a sort of "magical thinking" that goes beyond mere wishful thinking. In our need to make sense of the world, humans often grab hold of certain ideas and cling tight, even when those ideas may not be true and may not, in the end, serve us or the goals we are trying to reach. Human exceptionalism is one form of magical thinking, but even those who reject it are not immune from the pull of such thinking. Many social change activists are especially prone to magical thinking – they want so much to be righteous, they believe so deeply in their righteousness, that they think whatever they do must be righteous. Social reformers are strong visionaries, they are courageous, committed, and compassionate, but they are also human beings with egos, insecurities, and "issues."

Epistemic humility and activism are not often found together, although it would be useful if they were more often. In the face of so much injustice, it is hard both to maintain passion and to be open to alternative ideas and strategies. But, I would suggest, cultivating reflection and openness may be more conducive to bringing about a world in which more beings are able to flourish. Developing an ethical practice of engaged empathy is one way to expand our understanding of our place in our social and natural worlds and help us to respond more effectively to the ethical claims of others. Engaged empathy helps us to focus attention on the experiences of other animals and to look more closely at the features of their situations that threaten their well-being or might enable their flourishing. We've done a bit of that in this book. But, many of us are at some distance from animal pain, distress, fear, confusion, and suffering as well as from their joy, laughter, and contentment; other animals are abstractions – "chimpanzees" or "elephants" rather than Milla or Shirley. One way we might overcome this distance is to seek to connect with other animals, to volunteer at a shelter or a sanctuary, to "adopt" an animal in sanctuary and follow her development and experiences, to learn about animal behavior, to befriend other animals, maybe even fall in love with one (or more). Empathetic engagement with other animals is a form of moral attention that enhances our awareness of the claims they make on us, helps us to reorient our ethical sensibilities, and calls on us to exercise our moral agency. They need us to develop creative, compassionate, and ethical responses to them, for their sake as well as for our own.

References

Adams, Carol. 1990. *The Sexual Politics of Meat*. New York: Continuum.

2004. *The Pornography of Meat*. New York: Continuum.

Adelman, Jacob. 2009. "Mobile Slaughterhouse Assists in Trend to Locally Killed Meat." July 25. www.gosanangelo.com/news/2009/jul/25/mobile-slaughterhouse-assists-in-trend-to-killed/.

Allen, Colin. 1999. "Animal Concepts Revisited: The Use of Self-Monitoring as an Empirical Approach." *Erkenntnis*. Vol. 51 No. 1: 33–40.

American Academy of Physical Medicine and Rehabilitation. 2006. "Stem Cell Research and Therapy Proves Problematic for Rehabilitation Patients." www.aapmr.org/media/stemcell1106.htm.

Anderson, Elizabeth. 2004. "Animal Rights and the Values of Nonhuman Life." In Cass R. Sunstein and Martha Nussbaum (eds.). *Animal Rights: Current Debates and New Directions*. Oxford University Press: 277–98.

Animal Testing – Monkeys, Rats and Me. 2006. Television broadcast. BBC2. November 27. www.archive.org/details/MonkeysRatsandMe.

Arluke, Arnold, Frost, Randy, Steketee, Gail, Patronek, Gary, Luke, Carter, Messner, Edward, Nathanson, Jane, and Papazian, Michelle. 2002. "Press Reports of Animal Hoarding." *Society & Animals*. Vol. 10 No. 2: 113–35.

Aydede, Murat (ed.). 2006. *Pain: New Essays on its Nature and the Methodology of its Study*. Cambridge, Mass.: MIT Press.

Baden, John A. 1999. "Factory Farms Efficiency Comes with a High Price." *Bozeman Daily Chronicle*. January 20. www.free-eco.org/articleDisplay.php?id=187.

Barrett, Larry. 2002a. "From Egg to Drummies: 10 Weeks from Farm to Food." *Baseline Magazine*. July 10. www.baselinemag.com/c/a/Past-News/From-Egg-to-Drummies-10-Weeks-From-Farm-to-Food/.

2002b. "Poultry Production, Past and Present." *Baseline Magazine*. July 10. www.baselinemag.com/c/a/Past-News/Poultry-Production-Past-and-Present.

Bateson, Patrick. 1991. "Are There Principles of Behavioural Development?" In P. Bateson (ed.). *The Development and Integration of Behaviour: Essays in Honour of Robert Hinde*. Cambridge University Press.

Bekoff, Marc. 2002. *Minding Animals: Awareness, Emotions, and Heart*. New York: Oxford University Press.

2009. "Animal Emotions: Do Animals Think and Feel?" *Psychology Today*. www.psychologytoday.com/blog/animal-emotions/200906/wild-justice-and-moral-intelligence-in-animals.

Bekoff, Marc, and Pierce, Jessica. 2009. *Wild Justice: The Moral Lives of Animals*. The University of Chicago Press.

Bentham, Jeremy. 1789. "Of the Limits of the Penal Branch of Jurisprudence." *An Introduction to the Principles of Morals and Legislation*. London.

Berry, Colin, Patronek, Gary, and Lockwood, Randall. 2005. "Long-term Outcomes in Animal Hoarding Cases." *Animal Law*. Vol. 11: 167–88.

Biello, David. 2007. "Requiem for a Freshwater Dolphin." *Scientific American*. August 8. www.scientificamerican.com/article.cfm?id=requiem-for-a-freshwater-dolphin.

Bittman, Mark. 2008. "Rethinking the Meat-Guzzler." *New York Times*. January 27. www.nytimes.com/2008/01/27/weekinreview/27bittman.html.

Bjugstad, Kimberly B., Redmond, D. Eugene, Teng, Yang D., Elsworth, J. D., Roth, R. H., Blanchard, B. C., Snyder, Evan Y., and Sladek, John R. 2005. "Neural Stem Cells Implanted into MPTP-treated Monkeys Increase the Size of Endogenous Tyrosine Hydroxylase-positive Cells Found in the Striatum: A Return to Control Measures." *Cell Transplantation*. Vol. 14 No. 10: 183–92.

Boesch, Christophe, and Boesch, Hedwige. 1990. "Tool Use and Tool Making in Wild Chimpanzees." *Folia Primatologica*. Vol. 54: 86–99.

Boesch, Christophe, Bolé, Camille, Eckhardt, Nadin, and Boesch, Hedwige. 2010. "Altruism in Forest Chimpanzees: The Case of Adoption." *PLoS ONE*. Vol. 5 No. 1: e8901.

Boyd, William. 2001. "Making Meat: Science, Technology, and American Poultry Production." *Technology and Culture*. Vol. 42 No. 4: 631–64.

Bradshaw, Gay A. 2009. *Elephants on the Edge: What Animals Teach Us about Humanity*. New Haven, Conn.: Yale University Press.

Bradshaw, Gay R., Schore, Allan N., Brown, Janine L., Poole, Joyce H., and Moss, Cynthia J. 2005. "Elephant Breakdown." *Nature*. Vol. 433 No. 7028. February 24: 807.

Branch, John. 2010. "Where Creativity Wags its Tail." *New York Times*. April 18. www.nytimes.com/2010/04/19/sports/19grooming.html.

Broom, D. M., Sena, H., and Moynihan, K. L. 2009. "Pigs Learn What a Mirror Image Represents and Use it to Obtain Information." *Animal Behaviour*. Vol. 78 No. 5: 1037–41.

Brosnan, Sarah F., and de Waal, Frans B. M. 2002. "A Proximate Perspective on Reciprocal Altruism." *Human Nature*. Vol. 13 No. 1: 129–52.

Brown, James H., and Sax, Dov F. 2004. "An Essay on Some Topics Concerning Invasive Species." *Austral Ecology*. Vol. 29: 530–6.

Buckley, R. 2001. "Environmental Impacts." In David B. Weaver (ed.). *The Encyclopedia of Ecotourism*. New York: CABI: 379–90.

Caldwell, Mark. 2000. "Polly Wanna Ph.D.?" *Discover Magazine*. January 1. http://discovermagazine.com/2000/jan/featpolly.

Callicott, J. Baird. 1980. "Animal Liberation: A Triangular Affair." *Environmental Ethics*. Vol. 2 No. 4: 311–38.

    1989. *In Defense of the Land Ethic: Essays in Environmental Philosophy*. Albany, NY: SUNY Press.

Carlsson, Hans-Erik, Schapiro, Steven J., Farah, Idle, and Hau, Jann. 2004. "Use of Primates in Research: A Global Overview." *American Journal of Primatology*. Vol. 63 No. 4: 225–37.

Carvajal, Doreen, and Castle, Stephen. 2009. "A US Hog Giant Transforms Eastern Europe." *New York Times*. May 6. www.nytimes.com/2009/05/06/business/global/06smithfield.html.

Cataldi, Susan. 2002. "Animals and the Concept of Dignity: Critical Reflections on a Circus Performance." *Ethics and the Environment*. Vol. 7 No. 2: 104–26.

Chang, Ruth (ed.). 1997. Introduction. *Incommensurability, Incomparability and Practical Reason*. Cambridge, Mass.: Harvard University Press.

Chomsky, Noam. 1980. "Human Language and Other Semiotic Systems." In Thomas A. Sebok and Jean Umiker-Sebok (eds.). *Speaking of Apes: A Critical Anthology of Two-way Communication with Man*. New York: Plenum Press.

Christman, John. 2009. "Autonomy in Moral and Political Philosophy." *Stanford Encyclopedia of Philosophy*. http://plato.stanford.edu/entries/autonomy-moral/.

Clarke, Stephen R. L. 1977. *The Moral Status of Animals*. Oxford University Press.

Clayton, N. S., Bussey, T. J., and Dickinson, A. 2003. "Can Animals Recall the Past and Plan for the Future?" *National Review of Neuroscience*. Vol. 4: 685–91.

Clayton, N. S., and Dickinson, A. 1998. "Episodic-like Memory during Cache Recovery by Scrub Jays." *Nature*. Vol. 395 No. 117: 272–4.

Clayton, N. S., Salwiczek, L. H., and Dickinson, A. 2007. "Episodic Memory." *Current Biology*. Vol. 17 No. 6: R189–R191.

Clyne, Catherine. 2005. "(R)Evolution from Within? New Directions for the Humane Society: The *Satya* Interview with Wayne Pacelle." *Satya*. June/July. www.satyamag.com/jun05/pacelle.html.

Cochrane, Alasdair. 2009. "Do Animals Have an Interest in Liberty?" *Political Studies*. Vol. 57 No. 3: 660–79.

Cone, Tracie. 2009. "Calif. Lawmakers Rally Around Animal Welfare." *Associated Press*. May 29. www.bakersfieldnow.com/news/local/46501372.html.

"Conservationists Celebrate Double Achievement." 2008. *University of Kent*. September 18. www.kent.ac.uk/news/stories/conservationistsdoubleachievement/2008.

Convention on Biological Diversity. 2010. *Global Biodiversity Outlook 3*. www.cbd.int/GBO3.

Cook, John. 2006. "Thugs for Puppies." *Salon Magazine*. February 7. www.salon.com/life/feature/2006/02/07/thugs_puppies.

Cook, Michael. 1998. US House of Representatives Committee on Agriculture Hearing Statement. May 13. www.epa.gov/ocir/hearings/testimony/105_1997_1998/051398.htm.

Cripps, Elizabeth. 2010. "Saving the Polar Bear, Saving the World: Can the Capabilities Approach Do Justice to Humans, Animals and Ecosystems?" *Res Publica*. Vol. 16 No. 1: 1–22.

Cronin, William. 1996a. "Getting Back to the Wrong Nature: Why We Need to End our Love Affair with the Wilderness." *Utne Reader*. May/June. www.utne.com/1996–05-01/Environment/GettingBacktotheWrongNature.aspx?page=3.

    1996b. *Uncommon Ground: Rethinking the Human Place in Nature*. New York: W. W. Norton & Co.

Cuomo, Chris. 1998. *Feminism and Ecological Communities: An Ethic of Flourishing*. New York: Routledge.

Cuomo, Chris, and Gruen, Lori. 1998. "On Puppies and Pussies: Animals, Intimacy, and Moral Distance." In A. Bar-On and Ann Ferguson (eds.). *Daring to be Good: Essays in Feminist Ethio-politics*. New York: Routledge: 129–42.

Curtin, Deane. 1991. "Toward an Ecological Ethic of Care." *Hypatia*. Vol. 6: 60–74.

Cushman, Fiery. 2006. "Aping Ethics: Behavioral Homologies and Nonhuman Rights." In Marc Hauser, Fiery Cushman, and Matthew Kamen (eds.). *People, Property or Pets?* West Lafayette, Ind.: Purdue University Press.

Darwin, Charles. 1888. *The Descent of Man*. 2nd edn. London: John Murray. Vol. I.

Davenport, R. K., Jr., and Menzel, E. W. 1963. "Stereotyped Behavior of the Infant Chimpanzee." *Archives of General Psychiatry*. Vol. 8 No. 1: 99–104.

Davenport, R. K., Jr., Menzel, E. W., Jr., and Rogers, C. M. 1966. "Effects of Severe Isolation on 'Normal' Juvenile Chimpanzees: Health, Weight Gain, and Stereotyped Behaviors." *Archives of General Psychiatry*. Vol. 14 No. 2: 134–8.

Davidson, Donald. 1999. "The Emergence of Thought." *Erkenntnis*. Vol. 51: 7–17.

DeGrazia, David. 1996. *Taking Animals Seriously*. Cambridge University Press.

Department of Health and Human Services. 2005. Center for Disease Control and Prevention. "National Antimicrobial Resistance Monitoring System (NARMS)

Frequently Asked Question about Antibiotic Resistance." www.cdc.gov /narms/faq_antiresis.htm.

de Waal, Frans B. M. 2000. "Primates – A Natural Heritage of Conflict Resolution." *Science*. Vol. 289 No. 5479: 586–90.

Diamond, Cora. 1978. "Eating Meat and Eating People." *Philosophy*. Vol. 53 No. 206. October: 465–79.

2001. *The Realistic Spirit*. Cambridge, Mass.: MIT Press.

Donovan, Josephine. 1990. "Animal Rights and Feminist Theory." *Signs*. Vol. 15 No. 2: 350–75.

Donovan, Josephine, and Adams, Carol (eds.). 2007. *The Feminist Care Tradition in Animal Ethics*. New York: Columbia University Press.

Dorsey, E. R., Constantinescu, R., Thompson, J. P., Biglan, K. M., Holloway, R. G., Kieburtz, K., Marshall, F. J., Ravina, B. M., Schifitto, G., Siderowf, A., and Tanner, C. M. 2007. "Projected Number of People with Parkinson Disease in the Most Populous Nations, 2005 through 2030." *Neurology*. Vol. 68 No. 5: 384–6.

Edington, J. M., and Edington, M. A. 1986. *Ecology, Recreation and Tourism*. Cambridge University Press.

Engber, Daniel. 2009a. "Me and My Monkey: The Confessions of a Reluctant Vivisector." *Slate Magazine*. June 5. www.slate.com/id/2219228.

2009b. "Pepper Goes to Washington." *Slate Magazine*. June 3. www.slate.com /id/2219226/.

Environmental Integrity Project. 2008. "A Holiday Gift for Big Poultry Bush Administration Rushes Emissions Reporting Exemption." *Report of the Environmental Integrity Project*. December 9.

Etter, Lauren. 2008. "Have Knife, Will Travel: A Slaughterhouse on Wheels 'Custom Butcher' Gives Small Farms New Option to Sell Local Produce." *Wall Street Journal*. September 5.

Everett, Jennifer. 2001. "Environmental Ethics, Animal Welfarism, and the Problem of Predation: A Bambi Lover's Respect for Nature." *Ethics and the Environment*. Vol. 6 No. 1: 42–67.

Falk, J. H., Reinhard, E. M., Vernon, C. L., Bronnenkant, K., Deans, N. L., and Heimlich, J. E. 2007. *Why Zoos and Aquariums Matter: Assessing the Impact of a Visit to a Zoo or Aquarium*. Silver Spring, Md.: Association of Zoos and Aquariums.

Fearn, Eva (ed.). 2010. "2010–2011 State of the Wild: A Global Portrait." *Wildlife Conservation Society*. Washington, DC: Island Press.

Fedigan, Linda. 1992. *Primate Paradigms: Sex Roles and Social Bonds*. The University of Chicago Press.

Fiala, Nathan. 2009. "How Meat Contributes to Global Warming." *Scientific American*. February 4.

Fischer, J., and Lindenmayer, D. B. 2000. "An Assessment of the Published Results of Animal Relocations." *Biological Conservation*. Vol. 96 No. 1. November: 1–11.

Fitzgerald, Deborah Kay. 2003. *Every Farm a Factory*. New Haven, Conn.: Yale University Press.

Fluck, David. 2010. "Giants of Savanna the Latest Evolution at Dallas Zoo." *Dallas Morning News*. May 23.

Fouts, Roger. 1998. *Next of Kin: My Conversations with Chimpanzees*. New York: Harper Paperbacks.

Francione, Gary L. 1996. *Rain Without Thunder: The Ideology of the Animal Rights*. Philadelphia, Pa.: Temple University Press.

2000. *Introduction to Animal Rights: Your Child or the Dog?* Philadelphia, Pa.: Temple University Press.

2008. "'Pets': The Inherent Problems with Domestication." *Opposing Views*. August 27. www.opposingviews.com/arguments/pets-the-inherent-problems-with-domestication.

Frankfurt, Harry G. 1971. "Freedom of the Will and the Concept of the Person." *Journal of Philosophy*. Vol. 68 No. 1: 15–20.

Frey, R. G. 2002. "Justifying Animal Experimentation." *Society*. Vol. 39 No. 6 September/October: 37–47.

Gaard, Greta (ed.). 1993. *Ecofeminism: Women, Animals, Nature*. Philadelphia, Pa.: Temple University Press.

2002. "Vegetarian Ecofeminism: A Review Essay." *Frontiers: A Journal of Women Studies*. Vol. 23: 117–46.

Gardner, R. Allen, and Gardner, Beatrix T. 1969. "Teaching Sign Language to a Chimpanzee." *Science*. Vol. 165: 664–72.

1980. "Comparative Psychology and Language Acquisition." In Thomas A. Sebok and Jean Umiker-Sebok (eds.). *Speaking of Apes: A Critical Anthology of Two-way Communication with Man*. New York: Plenum Press: 287–329.

1989. *Teaching Sign Language to Chimpanzees*. State University of New York Press.

Godfrey-Smith, Peter. 2009. *Darwinian Populations and Natural Selection*. Oxford University Press.

Goodall, Jane. 1964. "Tool-using and Aimed Throwing in a Community of Free-living Chimpanzees." *Nature*. Vol. 201. March: 1264–6.

1986. *The Chimpanzees of Gombe: Patterns of Behavior*. Cambridge: Belknap Press.

Goodman, Peter S. 1999. "An Unsavory Byproduct: Runoff and Pollution." *Washington Post*. August 1. www.washingtonpost.com/wp-srv/local/daily/aug99/chicken1.htm.

Goodpaster, Kenneth. 1978. "On Being Morally Considerable." *Journal of Philosophy*. Vol. 75: 308–25.

Gould, Stephen Jay. 1997. "Kropotkin Was No Crackpot." *Natural History*. Vol. 106. June: 12–21.

Grau, Christopher (ed.). 2005. *Philosophers Explore* The Matrix. New York: Oxford University Press.

Griffiths, Paul E. 2002. "What is Innateness?" *Monist*. Vol. 85 No. 1: 70–85.

    2004. "Instinct in the '50s: The British Reception of Konrad Lorenz's Theory of Instinctive Behavior." *Biology and Philosophy*. Vol. 19 No. 4: 609–31.

Griffiths, Paul E., Machery, Edouard, and Linquist, Stefan. 2009. "The Vernacular Concept of Innateness." *Mind & Language*. Vol. 24 No. 5: 605–30.

Gross, Charles. 1998. "Galen and the Squealing Pig." *Neuroscientist*. Vol. 4: 216–21.

Gruen, Lori. 1993. "Dismantling Oppression: An Analysis of the Connection Between Women and Animals." In Greta Gaard (ed.). 1993. *Ecofeminism: Women, Animals, Nature*. Philadelphia, Pa.: Temple University Press.

    2002. "Refocusing Environmental Ethics: From Intrinsic Value to Endorsable Valuations." *Philosophy and Geography*. Vol. 5 No. 2: 153–64.

    2004. "Empathy and Vegetarian Commitments." In Steve, F. Sapontzis (ed.). *Food for Thought: The Debate over Eating Meat*. New York: Prometheus: 284–94.

    2009. "Attending to Nature: Empathetic Engagement with the More Than Human World." *Ethics and the Environment*. Vol. 14: 23–38.

Gruen, Lori, Grabel, Laura, and Singer, Peter (eds.). 2007. *Stem Cell Research: The Ethical Issues*. New York: Wiley-Blackwell.

Gruen, Lori, and Weil, Kari. 2010. "Teaching Difference: Sex, Gender, Species." In M. DeMello (ed.). *Teaching the Animal*. New York: Lantern Books: 127–44.

Hadley, John. 2009. "Animal Rights Extremism and the Terrorism Question." *Journal of Social Philosophy*. Vol. 40 No. 3: 363–78.

Hails, Chris (ed.). 2008. *Living Planet Report 2008*. Gland: WWF International.

Hancocks, David. 2003. *A Different Nature: The Paradoxical World of Zoos and their Uncertain Future*. Los Angeles, Calif.: University of California Press.

Hanson, Elizabeth. 2002. *Animal Attractions: Nature on Display in American Zoos*. Princeton University Press.

Haraway, Donna. 2008. *When Species Meet*. Minneapolis, Minn.: University of Minnesota Press.

Hare, B., Call, J., Agnetta, B., and Tomasello, M. 2000. "Chimpanzees Know What Conspecifics Do and Do Not See." *Animal Behaviour*. Vol. 59: 771–86.

Hare, B., Call, J., and Tomasello, M. 2001. "Do Chimpanzees Know What Conspecifics Know?" *Animal Behaviour*. Vol. 61: 139–51.

Harlow, Harry. 1974. *Learning to Love*. New York: Aronson.

Harlow, Harry, and Harlow, M. K. 1962. "Social Deprivation in Monkeys." *Scientific American*. Vol. 207 No. 5: 136–46.

Harper, A. Breeze (ed.). 2010. *Sistah Vegan: Black Female Vegans Speak on Food, Identity, Health, and Society*. New York: Lantern Press.

Harsanyi, John C. 1977. "Morality and the Theory of Rational Behavior." *Social Research*. Vol. 44 No. 4: 623–57.

Hasan, Nurdin. 2010. "Elephant Murder Mystery Highlights Threat Faced by Animals in Aceh." *Jakarta Globe*. May 9. www.thejakartaglobe.com/news/elephant-murder-mystery-highlights-threat-faced-by-animals-in-aceh/374091.

Hatkoff, Craig, Kahumbu, Isabelle, and Kahumbu, Paula. 2007. *Owen and Mzee: The True Story of a Remarkable Friendship*. New York: Scholastic Books.

Hauser, Marc. 2000. *Wild Minds: What Animals Really Think*. New York: Henry Holt and Company.

Hendrickson, M., and Heffernan, W. 2007. "Concentration of Agricultural Markets." *National Farmers Union*. April. Greenwood Village, Colo. www.nfu.org/wp-content/2007-heffernanreport.pdf.

Herrnstein, R. J. 1979. "Acquisition, Generalization, and Discrimination Reversal of a Natural Concept." *Journal of Experimental Psychology: Animal Behavior Processes*. Vol. 5: 116–29.

Herrnstein, R. J., Loveland, D. H., and Cable, C. 1976. "Natural Concepts in Pigeons." *Journal of Experimental Psychology: Animal Behavior Processes*. Vol. 2: 285–302.

Hess, Elizabeth. 2008. *Nim Chimpsky: The Chimp Who Would be Human*. New York: Bantam.

Heyes, C. M. 1998. "Theory of Mind in Nonhuman Primates." *Behavioral and Brain Sciences*. Vol. 21: 101–14.

Hockings, Kimberley J., Anderson, James R., and Matsuzawa, Tetsuro. 2006. "Road Crossing in Chimpanzees: A Risky Business." *Current Biology*. Vol. 16: R668–R670.

Horner, Victoria, and de Waal, Frans B. M. 2009. "Controlled Studies of Chimpanzee Cultural Transmission." *Progress in Brain Research*. Vol. 178: 3–15.

Horner, Victoria, Whiten, Andrew, Flynn, Emma, and de Waal, Frans B. M. 2006. "Faithful Replication of Foraging Techniques along Cultural Transmission Chains by Chimpanzees and Children." *Proceedings of the National Academy of Sciences*, 103: 13878–83.

House of Representatives. 2009. House Resolution 1549. "Preservation of Antibiotics for Medical Treatment Act." www.govtrack.us/congress/billtext.xpd?bill=h111-1549.

Hundley, Tom. 2005. "Village in Poland Clashes with US Pork Giant." *Chicago Tribune*. February 7.

Hunt, G. R. 1996. "Manufacture and Use of Hook-tools by New Caledonian Crows." *Nature*. Vol. 297: 249–51.

Hursthouse, Rosalind. 2000. *Ethics, Humans and Other Animals*. London: Routledge.

Hutchins, Michael, and Keele, Mike. 2006. "Elephant Importation from Range Countries: Ethical and Practical Considerations for Accredited Zoos." *Zoo Biology*. Vol. 25: 219–33.

Jamieson, Dale. 2002. *Morality's Progress: Essays on Humans, Other Animals, and the Rest of Nature*. Oxford University Press.

2008. *Ethics and the Environment*. Cambridge University Press.

Jeffries, Stuart. 2006. "Test Driven." *Guardian*. Interview. March 4. www.guardian .co.uk/animalrights/story/0,,1723372,00.html.

Johnson, George. 1995. "Chimp Talk Debate: Is it Really Language?" *New York Times*.

Kant, Immanuel. 1785. *The Groundwork for the Metaphysics of Morals*. Ed. and trans. Allen Wood. New Haven, Conn.: Yale University Press. 2002.

1798. *Anthropology from a Pragmatic Point of View*. Ed. and trans. Mary Gregor. The Hague: Martinus Nijhoff. 1974.

2001. *Lectures on Ethics*. Ed. J. B. Schneewind. Trans. Peter Heath. New York: Cambridge University Press.

Kawall, Jason. 1998. "Environmental Diversity and the Value of the Unusual." *Proceedings of the 20th World Congress of Philosophy*. www.bu.edu/wcp/Papers /Envi/EnviKawa.htm.

Keiger, Dale. 2009. "Farmacology." *Johns Hopkins Magazine*. Vol. 61 No. 3. www.jhu .edu/jhumag/0609web/farm.html.

Kellogg, W. N., and Kellogg, L. A. 1933. *The Ape and the Child*. New York and London: McGraw-Hill.

Kessler, M. J., Turnquist, J. E., Pritzker, K. P. H., and London, W. T. 1986. "Reduction of Passive Extension and Radiographic Evidence of Degenerative Knee Joint Diseases in Cage-raised and Free-ranging Aged Monkeys *(Macaca mulatta)*." *Journal of Medical Primatology*. Vol. 15: 1–9.

Kheel, Marti. 2008. *Nature Ethics: An Ecofeminist Perspective*. Lanham, Md.: Rowman & Littlefield.

Kittay, Eva. 2005. "At the Margins of Moral Personhood." *Ethics*. Vol. 116: 100–31.

2009. "The Personal is Philosophical is Political: A Philosopher and Mother of a Cognitively Disabled Person Sends Notes from the Battlefield." *Metaphilosophy*. Vol. 40 Nos. 3–4: 606–27.

Klailova, Michelle, Hodgkinson, Chloe, and Lee, Phyllis C. 2010. "Behavioral Responses of One Western Lowland Gorilla *(Gorilla gorilla gorilla)* Group at Bai Hokou, Central African Republic, to Tourists, Researchers and Trackers." *American Journal of Primatology*. April: 1–10.

Kluger, Jeffrey. 2007. "What Makes Us Moral?" *Time Magazine*. November 21.

Korsgaard, Christine. 1996. *The Sources of Normativity*. Cambridge University Press.

2004. "Fellow Creatures: Kantian Ethics and Our Duties to Animals." In Grethe B. Peterson (ed.). *The Tanner Lectures on Human Values*. Vols. 25–26. Salt Lake City, Utah: University of Utah Press.

2007. "Facing the Animal You See in the Mirror." Manuscript.

Krajick, Kevin. 2005. "Winning the War Against Island Invaders." *Science*. Vol. 310 No. 5753. December: 1410–13.

Kristof, Nicholas D. 2008. "A Farm Boy Reflects." *New York Times*. July 31.

2009. "Humanity Even for Nonhumans." *New York Times*. April 9.

Lederer, S. 1992. "Political Animals: The Shaping of Biomedical Research Literature in Twentieth-century America." *Isis*. Vol. 83 No. 1. March: 61–79.

Leider, J. P. 2006. "Animal Rights Activist Peter Singer Explains his Views." *Minnesota Daily*. March 23.

Lenman, James. 2000. "Consequentialism and Cluelessness." *Philosophy and Public Affairs*. Vol. 29 No. 4: 342–70.

Lewis, John. 2005. *US Senate Committee on Environment and Public Works Hearing Statements*. May 18. http://epw.senate.gov/hearing_statements.cfm?id=237817.

Lieberman, Bruce S., and Vrba, Elisabeth S. 2005. "Stephen Jay Gould on Species Selection: 30 Years of Insight." *Paleobiology*. Vol. 31 No. 2: 113–21.

Lindberg, K. 2001. "Economic Impacts." In David B. Weaver (ed.). *The Encyclopedia of Ecotourism*. New York: CABI: 363–75.

Lloyd, Elisabeth. 2004. "Kanzi, Evolution, and Language." *Biology and Philosophy*. Vol. 19 No. 4: 577–88.

Locke, John. 1690. *Essay on Human Understanding*. London.

Lockwood, Michael. 1979. "Singer on Killing and the Preference for Life." *Inquiry*. Vol. 22. Summer: 157–70.

Luban, Daniel. 2009. "Human Dignity, Humiliation and Torture." *Kennedy Institute of Ethics Journal*. Vol. 19 No. 3: 211–30.

Lusk, Jayson L. 2010. "The Effect of Proposition 2 on the Demand for Eggs in California." *Journal of Agricultural & Food Industrial Organization*. Vol. 8 No. 1.

Lyn, Heidi. 2007. "Mental Representation of Symbols as Revealed by Vocabulary Errors in Two Bonobos (*Pan paniscus*)." *Animal Cognition*. Vol 10: 461–75.

Mackenzie, Catriona, and Stoljar, Natalie (eds.). 2000. *Relational Autonomy: Feminist Perspectives on Autonomy, Agency, and the Social Self*. New York: Oxford University Press.

Mann, Janet, Sargeant, Brooke L., Watson-Capps, Jana J., Gibson, Quincy A., Heithaus, Michael R., Connor, Richard C., and Patterson, Eric. 2008. "Why Do Dolphins Carry Sponges?" *PLoS ONE*. Vol. 3 No. 12: e3868.

Marino, Lori, Lilienfeld, Scott O., Malamud, Randy, Nobis, Nathan, and Broglio, Ron. 2010. "Do Zoos and Aquariums Promote Attitude Change in Visitors? A Critical Evaluation of the American Zoo and Aquarium Study." *Society and Animals*. Vol. 18: 126–38.

McGowan, Christopher. 1997. *The Raptor and the Lamb: Predators and Prey in the Living World*. New York: Henry Holt and Company.

McMahan, Jeff. 2005. "Our Fellow Creatures." *Journal of Ethics*. Vol. 9: 353–80.

2008. "Eating Animals the Nice Way." *Daedalus*. Winter: 66–76.

Mellon, Margaret, Benbrook, Charles, and Benbrook, Karen Lutz. 2001. *Hogging It! Estimates of Antimicrobial Abuse in Livestock*. Cambridge, Mass.: Union of Concerned Scientists.

Meyers, Diana Tietjens. 2000. "Intersectional Identity and the Authentic Self? Opposites Attract!" In Catriona Mackenzie and Natalie Stoljar (eds.). *Relational Autonomy: Feminist Perspectives on Autonomy, Agency, and the Social Self*. New York: Oxford University Press.

Midgley, Mary. 1983. *Animals and Why They Matter*. Harmondsworth: Penguin.

Mill, John Stuart. 1859. *On Liberty*. London.

Mills, Brett. 2010. "Television Wildlife: Documentaries and Animals' Right to Privacy." *Continuum: Journal of Media and Cultural Studies*. Vol. 24 No. 2: 193–202.

Mistichelli, J. M. 1985. "Baby Fae: Ethical Issues Surrounding Cross-species Organ Transplantation." *Scope Note*. No. 5: 1–19.

Morgan, K. N., and Tromborg, C. T. 2007. "Sources of Stress in Captivity." *Applied Animal Behaviour Science*. Vol. 102: 262–302.

Muller, M., and Mitani, J. C. 2005. "Conflict and Cooperation in Wild Chimpanzees." In P. J. B. Slater, J. Rosenblatt, C. Snowdon, T. Roper, and M. Naguib (eds.). *Advances in the Study of Behavior*. New York: Elsevier: 275–331.

Murphy, Timothy. 2004. *Case Studies in Biomedical Research Ethics*. Cambridge, Mass.: MIT Press.

Myers, Norman. 1979. *The Sinking Ark: A New Look at the Problems of Disappearing Species*. New York: Pergamon Press.

Napier, John. 1964. "The Locomotor Functions of Hominids." In S. Washburn (ed.). *Classification and Human Evolution*. London: Methuen.

National Research Council. 2009. *Recognition and Alleviation of Pain in Laboratory Animals*. Washington, DC: The National Academic Press.

Nicholl, Charles S., and Russell, Sharon. 2001. "A Darwinian View of the Issues Associated with the Use of Animals in Biomedical Research." In Ellen Frankel Paul, Jeffrey Paul, and Fred D. Miller Jr. *Why Animal Experimentation Matters: The Use of Animals in Medical Research*. New Brunswick, NJ: Transaction Publishers.

Norris, Scott. 2007. "Tiny 'Crow-Cams' Capture Tool Use in Wild Birds." *National Geographic News.* http://news.nationalgeographic.com/news/2007/10/071004-crows-tools.html.

Novak, Melinda A., and Suomi, Stephen J. 1988. "Psychological Well-being of Primates in Captivity." *American Psychologist.* Vol. 43 No. 10: 765–73.

Nozick, Robert. 1974. *Anarchy, State, and Utopia.* New York: Basic Books.

Nussbaum, Martha. 2000. *Women and Human Development.* Cambridge University Press.

2004. "Beyond Compassion and Humanity: Justice for Nonhuman Animals." In Cass R. Sunstein and Martha Nussbaum (eds.). *Animal Rights: Current Debates and New Directions.* Oxford University Press: 299–320.

2006a. *Frontiers of Justice: Disability, Nationality, and Species Membership.* Cambridge: Belknap Press.

2006b. "The Moral Status of Animals." *Chronicle of Higher Education.* Vol. 52: B6–B8.

Oakley, Page. 1949. *Man the Toolmaker.* London: British Museum of Natural History.

Oyama, Susan. 2007. "Changing the Game." http://biolinguagem.com/colaboradores/oyama_2007_changingthegame.pdf.

Pacheco, Alex, with Francione, Anna. 1985. "The Silver Spring Monkeys." In Peter Singer (ed.). *In Defense of Animals.* New York: Basil Blackwell: 135–47.

Pearce, Fred. 1999. "Crops Without Profit: Britain is Paying an Extraordinary Price for its Agriculture." *New Scientist.* December 18.

Pew Charitable Trust. 2008. "Industrial Farm Animal Production, Antimicrobial Resistance and Human Health." *Pew Charitable Trust Report.* January 30.

Pitcher, George. 1995. *The Dogs Who Came to Stay.* New York: Dutton.

Plumwood, Val. 1993. *Feminism and the Mastery of Nature.* New York: Routledge.

2000. "On Being Prey." *Utne Reader.* July/August. www.utne.com/2000-07-01/being-prey.aspx.

Pollan, Michael. 2006. *The Omnivore's Dilemma: A Natural History of Four Meals.* New York: Penguin.

Poole, Joyce, and Granli, P. 2008. "Mind and Movement: Meeting the Interests of Elephants." In D. Forthman, L. L. F. Kane, and P. Waldau (eds.). *An Elephant in the Room: The Science and Well Being of Elephants in Captivity.* North Grafton, Mass.: Tufts University.

Povinelli, D., Eddy, T., Hobson, R., and Tomasello, M. (1996). *What Young Chimpanzees Know about Seeing.* Monographs of the Society for Research in Child Development. Vol. 61(3).

Pozos, Robert S. 2003. "Nazi Hypothermia Research: Should the Data be Used?" In Thomas E. Beam, and Linette R. Sparacino (eds.). *Military Medical Ethics.* Vol. 2. Office of the Surgeon General, United States Army.

Preece, Rod, and Chamberlain, Lorna. 1993. *Animal Welfare and Human Values*. Waterloo, Ont.: Wilfrid Laurier University Press.

Premack, David, and Premack, Ann James. 1984. *The Mind of an Ape*. New York: W. W. Norton & Co.

Prince-Hughes, Dawn. 2004. *Songs of the Gorilla Nation: My Journey through Autism*. New York: Harmony Books.

Pruetz, J. 2007. "Chimps Make and Use 'Spears' to Hunt." *National Geographic News*. http://news.nationalgeographic.com/news/2007/02/070222-chimp-video.html.

Pruetz, J., and Bertolani, P. 2007. "Savanna Chimpanzees, *Pan troglodytes verus*, Hunt with Tools." *Current Biology*. Vol. 17 No. 5: 412–17.

Redmond, D. Eugene, Jr. 2008. "Translational Studies in Monkeys of Human Embryonic Stem Cells for Treatment of Parkinson's Disease." *2008 Stem Cell Grants-in-Aid: Project Summaries and Updates*.

Reese, Jennifer. 2009. "What I Learned When I Killed a Chicken: Nothing Especially Virtuous." September 17. www.doublex.com/section/life/what-i-learned-when-i-killed-chicken.

Regan, Tom. n.d. "The Philosophy of Animal Rights." www.cultureandanimals.org/pop1.html.

1985. "The Case for Animal Rights." In P. Singer (ed.). *In Defense of Animals*. New York: Basil Blackwell: 13–26.

2001. *Defending Animal Rights*. Chicago, Ill.: University of Illinois Press.

2004. *The Case for Animal Rights*. Berkeley, Calif.: University of California Press.

Reiss, Diana, and Marino, Lori. 2001. "Mirror Self-recognition in the Bottlenose Dolphin: A Case of Cognitive Convergence." *Proceedings of the National Academy of Sciences*. Vol. 98 No. 10: 5937–42.

Roach, John. 2007. "Chimps Use 'Spears' to Hunt Mammals, Study Says." *National Geographic News*. http://news.nationalgeographic.com/news/2007/02/070222-chimps-spears.html.

Robinson, Phillip. 2004. *Life at the Zoo*. New York: Columbia University Press.

Rollins, Bernard E. 2006. "The Regulation of Animal Research and the Emergence of Animal Ethics: A Conceptual History." *Theoretical Medicine and Bioethics*. Vol. 27: 285–304.

Rolston, Holmes, III. 1988. *Environmental Ethics: Duties to and Values in the Natural World*. Philadelphia, Pa.: Temple University Press.

1994. *Conserving Natural Value*. New York: Columbia University Press.

Rosenthal, Elizabeth. 2010. "To Help Jaguars Survive, Ease their Commute." *New York Times*. May 11. www.nytimes.com/2010/05/12/science/earth/12jaguar.html?pagewanted=all.

Ross, S. R., Lukas, K. E., Lonsdorf, E. V., Stoinski, T. S., Hare, B., Shumaker, R., and Goodall, J. 2008. "Inappropriate Use and Portrayal of Chimpanzees." *Science*. Vol. 319: 1487.

Rudacille, Deborah. 2000. *The Scalpel and the Butterfly: The War Between Animal Research and Animal Protection*. New York: Farrar, Straus, and Giroux.

Rumbaugh, Duane M. 1980. "Language Behavior of Apes." In Thomas A. Sebok and Jean Umiker-Sebok (eds.). *Speaking of Apes: A Critical Anthology of Two-way Communication with Man*. New York: Plenum Press: 231–59.

Russell, Geoff, Singer, Peter, and Brook, Barry. 2008. "The Real Climate Change Culprit is Methane Gas from Cows and Sheep." *Melbourne Age*. July 10. www.theage.com.au/opinion/the-missing-link-in-the-garnaut-report-20080709 -3cjh.html?page= -1.

Sanz, Crickette M., Schöning, Caspar, and Morgan, David B. 2009. "Chimpanzees Prey on Army Ants with Specialized Tool Set." *American Journal of Primatology*. Vol. 71 No. 1: 1–8.

Savage-Rumbaugh, Sue, Shanker, Stuart G., and Taylor, Talbot, J. 1998. *Apes, Language and the Human Mind*. New York: Oxford University Press.

Schweitzer, Albert. 1936. "The Ethics of Reverence for Life." *Christendom*. Vol. 1: 225–39.

Sen, Amartya. 1992. *Inequality Reexamined*. Cambridge, Mass.: Harvard University Press.

Sensen, Oliver. 2009. "Kant's Conception of Human Dignity." *Kant-Studien*. Vol. 100 No. 3: 309–31.

Shapiro, Tamar. 1999. "What is a Child?" *Ethics* 109: 715–38.

Siddle, Sheila. 2002. *In My Family Tree: A Life with Chimpanzees*. New York: Grove Press.

Sidgwick, Henry. 1998. *Practical Ethics*. New York: Oxford University Press.

Singer, Peter (ed.). 1985. *In Defense of Animals*. New York: Basil Blackwell.

   1990. *Animal Liberation*. 2nd edn. New York: Avon Books.

   1993. *Practical Ethics*. Cambridge University Press.

Singer, Peter, and Mason, Jim. 2006. *The Way We Eat: Why Our Food Choices Matter*. Emmans, Pa.: Rodale Press.

Smith, Gavin J. D., Vijaykrishna, Dhanasekaran, Bahl, Justin, Lycett, Samantha J., Worobey, Michael, Pybus, Oliver G., Ma, Siu Kit, Cheung, Chung Lam, Raghwani, Jayna, Bhatt, Samir, Peiris, J. S. Malik, Guan, Yi, and Rambaut, Andrew. 2009. "Origins and Evolutionary Genomics of the 2009 Swine-origin H1N1 Influenza A Epidemic." *Nature*. Vol. 459: 1122–5.

Smithfield Foods. 2009. *Annual Report*. http://investors.smithfieldfoods.com /annuals.cfm.

Sorabji, Richard. 1993. *Animal Minds and Human Morals: The Origins of the Western Debate*. Ithaca, NY: Cornell University Press.

Spira, Henry. 1985. "Fighting to Win." In Peter Singer (ed.). *In Defense of Animals*. New York: Basil Blackwell: 194–208.

Steinfeld, Henning, Gerber, Pierre, Wassenaar, Tom, Castel, Vincent. Rosales, Mauricio, and de Hann, Cees. 2006. *Livestock's Long Shadow*. Rome: FAO.

Stevens, Christine. 1998. "Historical Motivation for the Federal Animal Welfare Act." In Michael Kreger, D'Anna Jensen, and Tim Allen (eds.). *Animal Welfare Act: Historical Perspectives and Future Directions*. www.nal.usda.gov/awic/pubs/96symp/awasymp.htm.

Strier, Karen. 2010. *The Challenge of Comparisons in Primatology*. http://onthehuman.org/2010/02/the-challenge-of-comparisons-in-primatology/.

Subak, Susan. 1999. "Global Environmental Costs of Beef Production." *Ecological Economics*. Vol. 30 No. 1: 79–91.

Suda-King, Chikako. 2008. "Do Orangutans (*Pongo pygmaeus*) Know When They Do Not Remember?" *Animal Cognition*. Vol. 11: 21–42.

Sugiyama, Y., and Koman, Jeremy. 1979. "Tool-using and -making Behavior in Wild Chimpanzees at Bossou, Guinea." *Primates*. Vol. 20: 513–24.

Taylor, A., Hunt, G., Holzhaider, J., and Gray, R. 2007. "Spontaneous Metatool Use by New Caledonian Crows." *Current Biology*. Vol. 17: 1504–7.

Taylor, Katy, Gordon, Nicky, Langley, Gill, and Higgins, Wendy. 2008. "Estimates for Worldwide Laboratory Animal Use in 2005." *Alternative to Laboratory Animals*. Vol. 36: 327–42.

Taylor, Paul. 1986. *Respect for Nature: A Theory of Environmental Ethics*. Princeton University Press.

Teichman, Jenny. 1985. "The Definition of Person." *Philosophy*. Vol. 60 No. 232: 175–85.

Terrace, H. S. 1983. "Apes Who 'Talk': Language or Projection of Language by their Teachers?" In Judith de Luce and Hugh T. Wilder (eds.). *Language in Primates: Perspectives and Implications*. New York: Springer-Verlag: 22–39.

Terrace, H. S., Petitto, L. A., Sanders, R. J., and Bever, T. G. 1979. "Can an Ape Create a Sentence?" *Science*. Vol. 206: 891–902.

Thorpe, W. H. 1950. "The Definition of Some Terms Used in Animal Behaviour Studies." *Bulletin of Animal Behavior*. 8: 34–50.

Tomasello, Michael, Call, Josep, and Hare, Brian. 2003. "Chimpanzees Understand Psychological States – The Question is Which Ones and to What Extent." *Trends in Cognitive Sciences*. Vol. 7: 153–6.

Tyson Foods, Inc. 2008. *Fiscal 2008 Fact Book*.

Union of Concerned Scientists. 2008. "CAFOs Uncovered: The Untold Costs of Confined Animal Feeding Operations." www.ucsusa.org/food_and_agriculture /science_and_impacts/impacts_industrial_agriculture/cafos-uncovered.html.

United States Department of Agriculture. 2008. "Environmental Interactions with Agricultural Production: Animal Agriculture and the Environment."

United States General Accounting Office. 2004. "Antibiotic Resistance: Federal Agencies Need to Better Focus Efforts to Address Risk to Humans from Antibiotic Use in Animals." *Report to Congressional Requesters*. Nos. 04–490. www.gao .gov/new.items/d04490.pdf.

VanDeVeer, Donald. 1979. "Interspecific Justice." *Inquiry*. Vol. 22: 55–79.

Van Minh, Tran. 2010. "Rare Rhino Shot, Horn Chopped, in Vietnam Preserve." *Associated Press*. May 10. http://abcnews.go.com/International/wireStory?id= 10602048.

Varner, Gary. 1998. *In Nature's Interests*. New York: Oxford University Press.

Vié, Jean-Christophe, Hilton-Taylor, Craig, and Stuart, Simon N. (eds.). 2009. *Wildlife in a Changing World: An Analysis of the 2008 IUCN Red List of Threatened Species*. Gland: IUCN.

Vierck, C. J., Hansson, P. T., and Yezierski, R. P. 2008. "Clinical and Pre-clinical Pain Assessment: Are We Measuring the Same Thing?" *Pain*. Vol. 135 Nos. 1–2: 7–10.

Walsh, Bryan. 2009. "America's Food Crisis and How to Fix it." *Time Magazine*. August 20. www.time.com/time/health/article/0,8599,1917458-1,00.html.

Warren, Samuel, and Brandeis, Louis. 1890. "The Right to Privacy." *Harvard Law Review*. Vol. 4 No. 5.

Watson, L. 2004. *The Whole Hog: Exploring the Extraordinary Potential of Pigs*. Washington, DC: Smithsonian Books.

Weir, A. A. S., Chappell, Jackie, and Kacelnik, Alex. 2002. "Shaping of Hooks in New Caledonian Crows." *Science*. Vol. 297 No. 5583: 981.

Weisman, Irving. 2005. "Chimeras: Animal–Human Hybrids." Interview with Tom Bearden. *News Hour*. August 16. www.pbs.org/newshour/bb/science/july-dec05 /chimera_ 8-16.html.

Wemmer, Christen, and Christen, Catherine A. 2008. *Elephants and Ethics: Toward a Morality of Coexistence*. Baltimore, Md.: Johns Hopkins Press.

Whiten, Andrew, Goodall, J., McGrew, W. C., Nishida, T., Reynolds, V., Sugiyama, Y., Tutin, C. E. G., Wrangham, R. W., and Boesch, C. 1999. "Cultures in Chimpanzees." *Nature*. Vol. 399: 682–5.

    2001. "Charting Cultural Variation in Chimpanzees." *Behaviour*. Vol. 138: 1481–516.

Whiten, Andrew, and Byrne, Richard. 1988. "Tactical Deception in Primates." *Behavioral and Brain Sciences*. Vol. 11 No. 2. June: 233–44.

Whiten, Andrew, Spiteri, Antoine, Horner, Victoria, Bonnie, Kristin E., Lambeth, Susan P., Schapiro, Steven J., and de Waal, Frans B. M. 2007. "Transmission of Multiple Traditions Within and Between Chimpanzee Groups." *Current Biology*. Vol. 17 No. 12: 1038–43.

Wilson, D. S. 1993. "Group Selection." In E. Keller and E. Lloyd, *Keywords in Evolutionary Biology*. Cambridge, Mass.: Harvard University Press: 145–8.

Wood, Allen. 1998. "Kant on Duties Regarding Nonrational Nature." *Proceedings of the Aristotelian Society*. Supplementary Vol. 72(1): 189–210.

Woodruff, Guy, and Premack, David. 1978. "Does the Chimpanzee Have a Theory of Mind?" *Behavioral and Brain Sciences*. Vol. 1: 515–26.

Woods, Vanessa. 2010. *Bonobo Handshake*. New York: Gotham Books.

Wuetrich, B. 2003. "Chasing the Fickle Swine Flu." *Science*. Vol. 299: 1502–5.

Wyse, Maureen. 2006. "Behind the SHAC: A Turning Point in Activism." *Satya*. December 2006–January 2007. www.satyamag.com/dec06/shac_intro.html.

Zimmer, Carl. 2007. "A Radical Step to Preserve a Species: Assisted Migration." *New York Times*. January 23.

Index